HOW CAN HELP YOU?

Information, Advice and Counselling for Gay Men and Lesbians

Malcolm Macourt was born in 1947 in Belfast and obtained his first degree at Birmingham University in 1968. After a year at a London college, he became a lecturer in economics at Dundee University. In 1973 he moved to Durham University where he was Fellow and Lecturer in Social Statistics in the North East Area Study Centre. He now teaches social research at Newcastle upon Tyne Polytechnic where he organises a specialist four-year honours degree in social research.

His experience as a volunteer counsellor involved with gay information, advice and counselling agencies is extensive. Since 1975 he has been a volunteer with FRIEND, the national gay befriending and counselling service. For three years he was a regional co-ordinator and for four years a member of the national management committee of National Friend Ltd, a registered charity, taking responsibility for monitoring the development of branches. He is now company secretary of National Friend Ltd. He has been involved in training on gay counselling methods for groups as diverse as police vice squads, the clergy and residential child care workers throughout the UK.

He was one of the research team responsible for the SIGMA projects, funded by the Department of Health and the Medical Research Council, which examined the impact of AIDS on the socio-sexual lifestyles of gay men.

His publications include *Towards a Theology of Gay Liberation* (SCM Press, 1977), which serves as a textbook in theological colleges on the gay issue from a radical liberal perspective.

HOW CAN WE HELP YOU?

Information, Advice and Counselling
for Gay Men and Lesbians

Malcolm Macourt

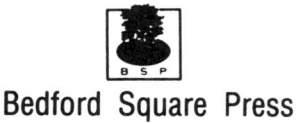

Bedford Square Press

Published by
Bedford Square Press of the
National Council for Voluntary Organisations
26 Bedford Square, London WC1B 3HU

First published 1989
© Malcolm P.A. Macourt, 1989

All rights reserved. No part of this publication may be reproduced or transmitted, in any form or by any means, electronic, mechanical, photocopying, recording or otherwise, without the prior permission of the publisher.

Typeset by The Word Shop, Rossendale, Lancashire
Printed and bound in England by Billing & Sons Ltd, Worcester

British Library Cataloguing in Publications Data

Macourt, Malcolm, *1947–*
   How can we help you? information, advice and counselling for gay men and lesbians.
   1. Great Britain. Homosexuality. Voluntary counselling organisations
   I. Title
   306.7'66'06041

ISBN 0–7199–1229–6

For Chris, Esme and Billy
and in memory of Frank

Contents

Acknowledgements	**ix**
Introduction	**xi**
What is a 'helpline'?	xi
What is a gay helpline?	xii
Why call them 'gay helplines'?	xiii
Scope of this book	xiv
1 The Development of Helplines	**1**
Why do helplines exist?	1
Why do gay helplines exist?	7
The development of gay helplines	10
Gay helplines in a typical region	16
Balancing influences	18
Summing up	21
2 Imagine You are a Volunteer and the Telephone Rings	**23**
Silence – 'What do I say?'	24
Confidentiality – 'Is anyone listening?'	27
Secrecy	28
Abusive calls	29
3 What Do Callers Ask?	**33**
'Am I gay/lesbian?'	33
'Will I get AIDS?'	39
'Where is the best gay pub in town?'	45
4 Being a Volunteer	**51**
Selection and training of volunteers	51
'Should I tell people what to do?'	60
'Can I answer anybody or only people like me?'	64

5 Callers and their World — 69
'Should I tell my parents?' — 69
'What about my marriage and my children?' — 74
'Should I be faithful to my lover?' — 78
'Will I fit into the gay world?' — 82

6 The More Difficult Problems — 91
'We have an odd one here – what do I do?' — 91
'How do I meet other transvestites?' — 99
'If you want a good time why telephone us?' — 103

7 Improving Helplines — 111
What functions do helplines have? — 111
Who else could provide these services? — 114
Assessing quality — 119
The birth, life (and death?) of helplines — 122
The future for gay helplines — 126

Notes — 129

Index — 143

Acknowledgements

Thanks are due to a large number of people for persuading me to write this book. First, to fellow volunteers in gay helplines, many of whom have been keen to see a book published which presents their experience and difficulties to a wider audience. Second, to those who have worked with me either as a volunteer during my 12 years with a gay helpline or as a member of the National Committee of FRIEND. Third, to those within the wider world of voluntary agencies, who persuaded me to link my gay helpline work to my work with other sorts of helplines.

When it came to the task of writing the book my thanks go, posthumously, to my long-time friend Frank Wilson, without whose encouragement the synopsis for this book would never have been written. Little did we know that nine months later he would have died as a result of AIDS. I hope that this book may be a fitting memorial to him.

In participating in a collective agreement whereby one of us is released from teaching duties in rotation, my colleagues in Applied Social Science at Newcastle upon Tyne Polytechnic assisted me.

My thanks are due to those who founded and developed gay helplines and particularly to those who inspired me through their writings, their leadership or their personal encouragement, particularly Jack Babuscio, Ted Clapham, Alison Hennigan, Stuart Hill, John Sketchley and Alan Swerdlow.

I owe a lot to my fellow volunteers, throughout the entire network of FRIEND helplines, but in particular to those who, like myself, have been involved in the work of FRIEND in the North East of England. I am grateful to those who have been responsible for co-ordinating that work at various times – Norman Powell, Keith Elliot, Derek Bodell, Eric Codling and Ann Widdas – and I am grateful to those national organisers with whom I have worked on the National Committee of FRIEND – Keith Hulbert, Margaret Gregory, Philip Conn and Norma Thompson.

Many people have spent a lot of time advising me on various sections of this book, but (at the risk of omitting important contributions) I particularly want to thank: Norma Thompson, Eric Codling, Sarah MacAdam, Paul Callender, Alex Mills, Maureen Gillman, Rory Murray and Michael Graham. Finally, without the care, encouragement and practical help of my friend Christopher Wardale the book would simply never have been completed.

Malcolm Macourt
August 1988

Introduction

What is a 'helpline'?

This book is about helplines – telephone-based services which provide information, advice and counselling to callers and it is about the volunteers who provide these services.

There are now a very large number of helplines of all sorts.[1]

Some of them are concerned with a particular group of people, some with a particular sort of problem, and some operate in a particular geographical area. Examples will be used from a variety of types of helpline because many of the problems of running helplines are common between different sorts of helpline.

However this book does have a particular focus. It is specifically about *gay helplines* – that is helplines which specialise in lesbian and gay issues.

In chapter 1, I describe some helplines, examine why they exist, and consider on what basis it is that they work. Chapters 2, 3, 4, 5 and 6 deal with the sorts of questions which are asked by callers, what these questions mean, what influences there are on each volunteer when answering them, and the problems faced by volunteers in working for a helpline and in answering the telephone. Many of these problems are common to volunteers on a wide variety of helplines.

First, in chapter 2, I look at issues which surround the start of each telephone call, silence, confidentiality and abuse.

Chapter 3 deals with the three most frequently asked questions – questions about personal identity, questions about fears of AIDS and HIV infection, and apparently simple requests for information.

In chapter 4 I look at life from the point of view of helpline volunteers, their selection and training, the amount of direct advice each one can and should give callers, and the issue of who it is may answer whom.

Chapter 5 considers issues concerning callers and their social environment, such as disclosure (to parents and to spouses in particular), relationships with lovers and fitting in to the gay social scene.

In chapter 6 several more difficult issues are considered, selected because they point to matters of principle involved in the work of the helplines.

Finally, in chapter 7, I ask and offer answers to the difficult questions 'how good are these helplines at helping their callers?' and 'how can the services offered be improved, if they need to be?'

Some helplines don't claim to provide counselling and advice, they claim to provide information alone. Many helplines do more than simply answer questions, they work with callers in other ways, through, for example, one-to-one meetings or drop-in centres or setting up self-help groups.

What is a gay helpline?

The total number of calls made each year to the 80 or so gay helplines in Great Britain and Ireland is approximately 400,000.[2]

The people who receive these calls claim to offer assistance. Making these calls are some people who simply want information, others who want a friendly chat, and more who are seeking advice on a serious personal problem, maybe about AIDS, or about family and relationships. Receiving these calls are gay men and lesbians who have volunteered for helpline work. What is different about gay helplines is the way which our society views lesbians and gay men, so that forms an important part of this book.

For the purposes of this book I shall define some helplines as *gay* helplines, to distinguish them from other helplines.

How am I limiting my use of the label 'gay helpline'? Whether they know it or not, all helplines from time to time deal with gay or lesbian callers. However, a 'gay helpline' is different in that it gears itself, either exclusively or primarily, towards those who are concerned about sexual relations between people of the same sex.

Also I am limiting my use of the label 'gay helpline' to those helplines which recognise that gay is good: that same-sex and opposite-sex relationships are of equal value, and neither is inferior to the other.

So I am not looking at the activities of certain 'new right', 'family life' or 'moral majority' groups, who operate what they claim to be telephone counselling services for 'those with a homosexual problem', since, even though they gear their service to gay men and lesbians, these organisations believe that gay is bad.[3]

Why call them 'gay helplines'?

In choosing the term *gay helpline* I am using a phrase which may need further explanation to two rather different groups of readers, those who feel ill at ease with the post-war use of the word 'gay', and those who prefer a term like 'lesbian and gay'.

Firstly, the term 'gay' is used throughout in preference to the term 'homosexual', since the latter term was an invention of the medical profession in the nineteenth century seeking to control same-sex activity.[4]

I do not wish to use a term with such clear implications of antagonistic social control.

The issue of the morality of same-sex relationships is considered in chapter 2. However, this book acknowledges the essential worth of all relationships. Just because a relationship is between two people of the same sex does not make it better or worse than a relationship between a man and a woman. Just because a man and a woman formalise their relationship by getting married does not make it any better than a relationship which does not enjoy such social, religious and legal approval.

Secondly, the term *gay helpline* may need explanation to those who now do not use the word 'gay' when referring to women as well as men. We have (rightly in my view) moved a long way in the words we use to describe proud, self-assured 'women-identified' woman and 'men-identified' men. We do not use 'homosexual' any more. In the last 10 years we have stopped using 'gay' as an umbrella word for both woman and men. We now use phrases like 'lesbians and gay men' or 'lesbian woman and gay men' when both groups need to be addressed together.

I have here used the phrase *gay helplines* for ease of expression only, and to avoid a more cumbersome phrase. This does not mean that I reject the language changes of the 1980s. Gay helpline is also used in a general sense to describe both those helplines which offer their services only to men or only to women.

There are gay helplines throughout Great Britain and Ireland.[5]

They use a variety of different names for the service they offer. The most frequent are: Lesbian and Gay Switchboard,

FRIEND, Gay Switchboard, Lesbian Line and Gayline.

This book focuses on the work of local and regional gay helplines, and in particular those within the federation of gay information, befriending and counselling services known as FRIEND.

Scope of this book

The experience and research on which this book is based does not include direct experience of working on lines other than mixed-sex gay helplines. So, for example, it does not include the work of any of the lesbian-only lines.[6]

It would be presumptuous for a man to be the author of a book which claimed to study women-only helplines, just as it would be presumptuous for a white person to be the author of a book which claimed to study helplines run by and for black people. However, I hope that some of the insights in this book may be of relevance to the operation of all helplines, but only those involved may judge.

Helplines: do they help their callers? If so, how and, if need be, how can that assistance be improved? These are the questions this book seeks to answer.

1 The development of helplines

Why do helplines exist?

Before we examine how helplines operate and how good they are, we need to establish what they are doing and why.

At one level helplines fulfil the role of the 'neighbour'. On occasions we all need a neighbour to whom we can turn, a neighbour who will lend us some sugar, with whom we can have a chat, or have a moan, a neighbour who will see us through a crisis.

The helpline may fulfil the role of the neighbour because the locality in which the caller lives does not work like that, or because the caller sees the problem as so enormous that it is not possible to involve someone they already know.

One essential part of the chat or the moan, or the request for advice from that neighbour, is that both my neighbour and I are part of the same community. We both share in its set of values. One of the things which we are doing when we seek advice from a neighbour is checking out what our shared values mean in a particular context. So the advice-seeker is checking out thoughts, feelings and proposed courses of action, to ensure that they are similar to what the neighbour would think, feel and propose to do in the same situation. The asking for, and giving of, advice confirms the values both share, and in the process comforts or improves the life of the seeker. Nothing more is attempted, nothing more is expected.

At another level a helpline is supplanting or supplementing the role of the professional adviser. Thirty years ago to seek advice normally meant consulting a doctor, a lawyer or a clergyman. He was male (almost without exception), he knew the answers to the questions you asked and you knew that you were expected to abide by the advice he gave.

All that has changed – in two ways. No longer does counselling happen when established professionals pronounce on the difficulties felt by the rest of us. Nowadays many professionals act in a different way towards their clients, working with them through the problems presented. Maybe the helpline, without claiming any status as a professional service, offers to serve by being available to them in times of trouble.

There has been a massive growth of advice services and helplines of many sorts. The growth in volunteer-staffed telephone helplines was most marked in the early 1980s, but older examples began their work in the 1950s.

The Samaritans

Perhaps the starting point of this development was the decision of a City of London vicar, Rev Chad Varah, to staff a telephone and invite those who felt suicidal to call.[1]

He, a professional, encouraged volunteers to staff the line with him. He gathered groups of people together to offer a service on a telephone. From that small beginning has grown the service, known as the Samaritans, which exists throughout the UK and which has links with similar services in many countries. The service which is offered fills gaps left from the partial collapse of close-knit communities, gaps which it seemed professional advisers were unable or unwilling to fill.

The Samaritans have had an important influence, both directly and indirectly, on all subsequent helplines.[2]

The working methods of the Samaritans have some parallels in many helplines: for example, a training programme for volunteers; anonymity of volunteers: and rules of procedure like 'never hang up on a caller'.

So some helplines are general in appeal and purely humanitarian in approach. This includes some which claim merely to provide information in an increasingly complex world. But most helplines have a particular focus – on a particular group of callers or a particular problem or issue – and a more specific set of objectives.

Providing help may merely maintain the existing social environment by easing the adjustment problems which some people present; or it may encourage people to empower themselves, that is to take control of and responsibility for their own future and to help them associate themselves with moves to restructure the existing social world, through assisting them with what they see to be their individual problems. Deliberately or not, most helplines try to help society change, as the following examples show.

A woman with cancer may be told how social services may help her, how to ensure that she may receive the best available NHS treatment, and may be helped to tell her family that her illness is terminal – all very praiseworthy and full of humanitarian concern – and/or she may be given information about alternative forms of health care, or about self-help groups designed to improve the self-esteem of women in her position, or she may be put in contact with those who are campaigning for further government resources for research into cancer.

A young Asian man, concerned about expectations about his involvement in an arranged marriage, may be helped work through his worries about his impending marriage, and/or he may be put in contact with those who share his racial and religious background who have found alternative lifestyles.

Put another way, a helpline may provide help which acts like sticking plaster in helping a cut to heal, or it may include advice which will help prevent recurrences of the cut, even to the extent of 'removing the knife'.

Advice is never neutral

Advice may support the social status quo or it may challenge it. Either way it may be well-intentioned or given with evil-intent. It may be lovingly given or given without proper care. Either way it may be given in a style which dictates or one which tries to avoid dictating. Either way the advice may be good advice or bad advice – it may be my advice (always good?) or someone else's advice (only sometimes good?). But whoever gives the advice, whatever style it is given in, with however good an intent, it is never neutral. Inevitably it represents something of the values of the advice-giver and of his or her view of the world we live in, and the contexts in which the advice-giving organisation works.

Social and political change

Given that advice is never neutral, should a helpline deliberately help society change? Should a helpline reflect existing society or should it promote change in the social order?

Should volunteers restrict themselves to helping callers with their immediate problems and try to minimise any desire they may have to change society?[3]

This debate has been ever-present in discussions among

helpline volunteers. 'We must not be political' has stood against 'We cannot be anything but political.'

There is no reason to be ashamed of being political if it is understood in the widest sense of the word. I define any activity as 'political' if it helps people draw conclusions about their own circumstances, if it helps them see that their own lives would be enhanced if (with others) they could change some aspect of the social order, and if it helps them find ways to effect such change.

So, for example: A helpline which helps people dominated by alcohol is being political if, in helping a caller, that caller comes to see that the unrecognised breakdown of her relationship with her husband has been a cause of her addiction to alcohol. The helpline is being political in that it is assisting callers to separate from their spouses, thereby working against declared government policy in defending family life.

A helpline which helps those with multiple sclerosis and their relatives and friends is being political if its callers come to realise that health and welfare facilities are inadequate or inappropriate. If the helpline provides its callers with information about ways to bring pressure on health or welfare authorities or government to make changes, it is being political.

Another way of looking at the matter of social and political change is to consider a helpline whose volunteers are devotees of a particular political or religious outlook and who see themselves as doing 'missionary' work when they are helpline volunteers.

Evangelising missionaries

Fringe cults have long used a wide variety of advertising techniques to 'sell' their particular political or religious outlook. A 'telephone ministry' can be one of these techniques.

Those who conduct political opinion polls or genuine market research interviews get very annoyed with sales personnel who misuse either street interview techniques or telephone interview techniques (which are superficially similar to their own) to sell products – 'SUGing' (selling under the guise of . . .) as it is known in the trade. In the same way volunteers on some helplines get very annoyed with the activities of 'missionary' helplines – those who wear their ideological hearts on their sleeves. However, we must not dismiss these helplines too quickly.

The 'missionary' helpline offers specific solutions to problems raised by callers. It ensures that volunteers assist callers towards those solutions which fit in with the missionary 'gospel', whatever it may be. The volunteer helps the caller to present his or her problems in such a way as to allow the caller to see the pertinence of the solutions which emerge from the 'gospel'.

For some readers examples of evangelising missionaries such as the Moonies will come to mind, for others examples such as Jerry Falwell (or other American Christian fundamentalists) will be uppermost, for others, perhaps, free-marketeers, for others Marxist-Leninists. What is seen as unacceptable evangelising depends on where the reader starts from, and therein lies the difficulty of analysing the work of these helplines. It is not easy to judge the extent to which each volunteer on each helpline sees a duty to 'sell' a particular ideology on the phone.

The boundary line between the selling of an ideology – 'evangelising' – and the caring for the callers is difficult to draw and grey areas are difficult to avoid. Even supposedly neutral helplines, such as the Samaritans, hold fast to a view of suicide – that it is to be avoided if at all possible – which can be seen as ideological.[4]

Perhaps that ideology is supported by the very vast majority of us, but it is not a value-free non-partisan position, it is an ideology. Perhaps it could be called Christian-inspired humanitarianism.

In this context, merely allowing (for example), a male caller to say that he feels happy to have sex with another man is seen by some people as unacceptably political because they see it as 'promoting homosexuality'. They consider it to be the duty of responsible persons to point out the intrinsic evil of such feelings, and the sin in such acts. To very many people, including volunteers on gay helplines, allowing the caller to speak in this way is commonplace and to think of it as political or ideological is ridiculous. So just as humanitarian concern can readily be seen as an influence on the practice of all helplines, so also each helpline will have ideals concerning the particular group or issue which is the primary focus of its work.

Whether they are dealing with those who have been recently bereaved, those who have spina bifida, or those whose origins are in a particular culture, helplines concerned with each group operate with a focus (or a political position, or an ideology – call it what you will) which furthers the best interests of their group of callers.

In each helpline a consensus emerges between humanitarian concern and the demand to serve the best interests of the group of callers.

A special world

However, there may be another influence which may have different consequences – the influence of the ghetto. Many groups in our society have created special worlds for themselves, special worlds separate from the unsavoury world of the detractors of the group – racists, homophobics, misogynists, those who despise the physically handicapped or the alcohol-dependent or whoever.

Each of us in our own way manages the world by living in only part of it, limiting our concerns to (for example) family, the workplace, the weather, the price of food and the annual Spanish holiday. If our 'little' world contains most of the ingredients for a form of happiness there seems little point in bothering to do anything about the 'bigger' world – either to engage with it or to change it. We must live in it but we can ignore it as far as possible.

This 'little' world consists of those around us – such as neighbours, family and friends. But if anything causes the little world to fall apart – such as being told that you have cancer, or (in some white circles) marrying a black person, or realising that you are gay or lesbian – then a new 'little' world may be immediately necessary, at least temporarily. The second half of the twentieth century has seen the broadening of the limited geographical basis of most 'little' worlds – but the cultural dimensions have remained almost intact – shared assumptions, dependance on the familiar, fear of the unknown or the unusual, trepidation and retrenchment when faced with rapid change.

What if you are the one whose 'little' world has fallen apart? Is it possible to create a new 'little' world to replace the old one? Plainly the answer is yes – there are those who live their lives (almost) entirely surrounded by those of like mind, or with shared characteristics of one type or another, all gay, all black, all people with multiple sclerosis.

So it is with helpline volunteers. Imagine a helpline whose volunteers all see themselves as belonging to a particular group of people who are maltreated, misunderstood or discriminated against by the rest of society. That group may be of people with a particular physical or mental ability or disability, or of people from a particular racial or religious environment, or of people who have had a particular life experience, for example those who have been raped or who have been recently bereaved.

Members of the group may be easily identifiable in the street, or they may be hidden from view. For each the discrimination felt may be all real or partly imagined. The discrimination may be clearly recognised for what it is, or it may have become internalised – for example in the gay male context it may be internalised as 'all gay men are no good, therefore I am no good'.

Volunteers in such a helpline would want to show the advantages to their own lives of belonging to the group. The callers could be assured that they were eligible for membership of the group. They could be persuaded that it is acceptable to be part of the group, and helped to identify with other members of the group. Two more examples may assist here.

How much of an advantage is it to the mother of a child who has recently died to introduce her to others who have been similarly bereaved? If it is of immediate benefit (as it may be), is it of long-term benefit for her to remain part of such a bereavement group? May not feelings of discrimination against the bereaved eventually be increased if she has not been allowed to work through her bereavement by dealing with her memories and placing them in a wider context?

The man who has spina bifida may benefit from seeing the achievements of others like himself, and may benefit from participating in seeking solutions to problems common to many others with spina bifida – but if his whole world revolves round others with spina bifida will he not suffer through long-term isolation from the wider world?

Each helpline balances the influences upon it, taking account of its historical development, its volunteers, its social environment and its callers. But most of all, it is affected by the social context in which it operates.

Why do gay helplines exist?

Turning now to the specific focus of this book, gay helplines, I want to consider why they came into existence, the social context in which they operate, and the changes there may have been since their founding.

Views about gay men and lesbians

Most people in Britain ignore gay and lesbian identities. Their views are ill-formed, being a mixture of mild distaste, a fear for children, and a desire to let people live their own lives in their own way. For them it is not an important issue.[5]

A minority, usually those with gay or lesbian friends or family members, actively support lesbians and gay men in their desire to live full and satisfying lives without fear and hatred. Often it *is* an important issue for them.

Another minority wish to destroy any form of positive gay or lesbian identity, wishing to continue to heap ridicule and humiliation on those who do not conform to their views of femininity and masculinity. Many in gay and lesbian circles hold that this minority include a lot of people who have gay or lesbian sexual identity but who reject that identity. The evidence for this view is considerable but inconclusive. Volunteers on gay helplines often find that (particularly) older callers eventually comment on their own virulent opposition before they plucked up courage to telephone a gay helpline to discuss their own identity. There is also much anecdotal evidence that many of the leaders of anti-gay attacks have a hidden gay identity perhaps known only to a small coterie of the like-minded. Most of the anecdotes concern the Church, the armed forces and Parliament.[6]

Another minority, comprising many gay men and lesbian women, but not all (see above), seek to enhance the views people have of gay and lesbian identity. They seek to protect themselves from attack – physical as well as verbal – and they seek to extend the positive changes which have occured in the last 25 years in enhancing the status of gay men and lesbians.

Advice for 'homosexuals'?

There are particular reasons why gay helplines have come into existence, reasons which play an important part in the development of a philosophical basis on which gay helplines operate, and so need to be examined carefully. The first of these reasons concerns the history of advice-giving relating to gay and lesbian matters.

Until the 1960s, almost the only advice for those who saw themselves as 'homosexual' was 'Don't do anything, try to overcome your problem.'[7]

Sexual abstinence was seen as the only acceptable solution to the 'problem' of 'homosexuality'. At that time 'homosexuality' was seen as a problem, and problems require solutions.

Since then changes in attitudes to sex have had an impact on the advice offered by professional advisers.[8] It is still not difficult to find clergy and psychiatrists who view gay or lesbian sexuality as a problem for the individual, but it is easier to find professionals who see it as a problem for society at large as well as for the individual. Many professions go much further. They see it as a problem for society alone.

Some have gone further still to rethink what a 'problem' is, and they now argue that to think in terms of a 'problem' at all is inappropriate. 'Problems' are those things which are inconvenient to those in control of our society and some professionals are now asking questions about who controls society and why.

Seeking advice about 'homosexuality' used to mean consulting a doctor or a minister of religion. He was male – almost certainly. He had to be heterosexual, or at least pretend to be so. For a professional advice giver to admit to homosexuality not only placed his professional career in jeopardy, it automatically removed validity from the advice being given. No one would have advised 'indulgence' in gay sexual identity, since that would have been seen as recruitment (to an evil cause). It seemed unimaginable that 'self-confessed homosexuals' would claim to advise other people with the same 'problem'.

The changing face of advice-giving

But now there are 80 or so volunteer telephone advice-giving agencies staffed almost exclusively by those self-same 'homosexuals', both male and female.[9] Now men and women volunteers who identify themselves as lesbian or gay listen carefully to callers, helping them from within their experience and expertise to make sense of their lives.

In addition to changes concerning advice giving, there are changes in our society which have helped change the environment for advice giving on gay or lesbian sexuality in the past 30 years. These changes are:

- A change in the place of women in society. However limited the extent of that change may seem, it has been profound.

No longer can it be assumed that the minister of religion, the doctor or the psychiatrist who offers the advice on sexuality will almost automatically be male – but the change is one of ethos, not merely a change in numbers. Middle-class professional men can no longer regard the world as a closed club run by and for its own members. That club has had its doors forced open, its constitution rewritten and it has lost much of its power and influence.

- A change in the feelings which lesbians and gay men have about individual and group worth.

The self-esteem of many gay men and lesbians has dramatically improved, often because people are able to identify with a group which has a positive identity. This change – which

I shall call 'empowerment' – has allowed them to stand up to exploitation both from without and within.

Perhaps the first public manifestation of this empowerment was in the movements which started in the early 1970s – the Gay Liberation Front and the Campaign for Homosexual Equality. First and foremost gay liberation declared the positive value of identifying with one's own sex and not just where it concerns same-sex sexual activity.[10] Early gay liberationists saw the need to challenge a social order which reduced 'homosexuals' to objects of humiliation or ridicule and which refused to permit the issue to be discussed. Gay liberationists saw links between the treatment of gay men and lesbians and the treatment of other 'oppressed' groups: lesbians first, women in general next, blacks and Asians, children, old people, people with mobility handicaps, with sensory handicaps, people with learning problems and many others.

For some gay liberationists there was a further and fundamental link, that between gay liberation and class. Some advocates of gay liberation saw the link between their oppression and the oppression of the working class, and so they sought to create alliances with supporters of Karl Marx and his followers in seeking to ensure a society free from all oppressions.[11]

The development of gay helplines

Many different factors influenced the formation of gay helplines, and this variety partly explains the diversity among them. The formal histories of the larger and better-known helplines have yet to be written but it is likely that those histories will focus on three factors, two of them specific to gay and lesbian matters.

Histories will focus on the development of a gay liberation philosophy in the United States in the late 1960s (which owed much to earlier and parallel liberation movements concerning blacks and women) and its arrival in Europe. Histories will also focus on the passing of the 1967 Sexual Offences Act which (for England and Wales) removed penalties from consenting sexual acts between two adult men in private.[12] Despite its many faults, this Act provided an environment in which gay liberation ideas could flourish. In addition, historians may take account of the emerging youth cultures of the 1960s and changes in the media and the impact of the 'underground' or 'alternative' society on the lives of young people at that time.

The early days – FRIEND and Gay Switchboards

In April 1971 the reformists of the gay world, the Campaign for Homosexual Equality (CHE), built into their constitution a requirement that advice and counsel be provided for those in need of it. It was soon realised that this activity needed to be separated from the run-of-the-mill social and political activities of the branches of CHE, so the advice and counselling arm was given a separate identity, and thereby FRIEND was founded. Initially FRIEND was a part of CHE, but operated entirely separately. In 1977 FRIEND completed the process of distancing itself from the campaigning role which CHE espoused.[13] The commitment which CHE made in 1971 carried on a tradition established in 1958 when members of the newly-founded Homosexual Law Reform Society set up the Albany Trust as its counselling arm, though the style and content of the exercise was rather different.[14] The Albany Trust sought to provide liberal advice through counselling sessions on a one-to-one basis or by letter, always retaining a certain distance between counsellors and the growing openly gay community. From the beginning, FRIEND, on the other hand, made its involvement with the gay community clear and conducted much of its activity by telephone using volunteers, very many of whom were avowedly gay or (in smaller numbers) lesbian.

In early 1973 one of the early gay liberation groups saw the need to facilitate the recruitment to their cause of those for whom 'homosexuality' remained a personal problem.[15] The London-based Icebreakers owed its origin to this group and the explicit gay liberation perspective remained with it throughout its existence as a telephone-based helpline. The idea of 'recruiting' people to a gay lifestyle may seem unusual. However, 'recruitment' is only viewed with suspicion when we view the cause which is doing the recruiting with suspicion. When the cause is a good one, recruiting people to it must also be good.

In 1974, a few years after the founding of FRIEND, what quickly became the largest of all the gay helplines was founded, London Gay Switchboard (which became London Lesbian and Gay Switchboard in 1984).[16] By that time, *Gay News*, which served from 1972 to the early 1980s as the major source of information on gay-related activities both of a political and a social nature, was already listing several dozen contact telephone numbers for information and advice.[17] These telephone numbers covered most of the major centres of population. Within a year or so many of these contact telephone numbers were describing themselves by names like 'Gay Switchboard'.

1974 – 1984

The next 10 years saw a general growth in gay helplines. Almost every major centre of population acquired one, then maybe a second as there was seen to be a need both for an information service (a Gay Switchboard) and a counselling and befriending service (a FRIEND group). Soon also the larger centres of population acquired a third (a Lesbian Line) as many women had found it too difficult to work in a predominately male environment, which often failed to recognise them, and had set up women-only lines.[18] All three types of helpline formed more or less close working arrangements.

In smaller centres the enthusiasm for a working helpline has often rested on very few volunteers. Many smaller centres have had a gay helpline for a while during the last 15 years, but not for all of the time. It is sometimes quite difficult to keep up with the numbers of small-town helplines which are opening and closing.

By 1979 most of the major gay helplines which now exist in regional centres had been founded in one form or another, so they have had at least a decade's experience.

1984 onwards: attacks – AIDS, Parliament and the Church

In the last five years there have been several developments which have had their effect on gay helplines.

AIDS

The period since the recognition of AIDS as a matter of grave concern to many gay men, and particularly the period since the beginning of the political backlash against gay men and lesbians, has found additional strains being placed on gay helplines. Not only are more and more people telephoning the helplines, but some helplines have experienced difficulties with recruitment as many potential volunteers devote their energies specifically to matters concerning AIDS and HIV infection and/or to more overtly political matters relating to the position of gay men and lesbians in society.

AIDS has provided an excellent opportunity for parts of the press to fan the flames of antagonism towards gay men.[19] In part the hysteria surrounding AIDS concerned fear of any new 'killer disease', but in large measure it concerned homophobia, an abnormal fear of 'homosexuality'.[20] Much of the early press comment on AIDS (continued sadly still by some papers) presented gay men as the perpetrators of AIDS rather than the sufferers from it.

Hysteria in society reached its peak in early 1985 when the press found that an Anglican clergyman, who was a prison chaplain, had died as a result of AIDS.[21] The press reports the following day, for example calling for the testing of all the prisoners in case he had had sex with them, made grizzly reading. No one seemed to care about the family and friends of the clergyman concerned.

The early response of many gay men to this renewed public hatred was to retreat still further from the public gaze (into 'the closet'). They admitted their sexual preference to fewer people, and moved closer to having two lives: one life in the office or on the shop floor with its (sometimes entirely fictitious) stories of wife and children, and another at home with a male lover and gay friends.

A few, a very few at the beginning, responded by redoubling their efforts to alter general perceptions of same-sex relations. The pattern in the UK mirrored the pattern in the USA where the AIDS phenomenon arrived a few years earlier – more fear, more retreats into 'the closet', but also more political activism.[22]

The increased activism, and widespread unease at the over-reaction of the media, has produced results. There had grown up a network of helplines specifically concerned with AIDS and Human Immuno-deficiency Viral (HIV) infection. The first of these, run by the Terrence Higgins Trust, began in 1984, and now there are over 20 AIDS lines which specialise in dealing with calls from gay men throughout the country.[23] These are staffed largely by gay men and lesbians. (This book does not concern itself in detail with AIDS lines, though much of it has direct relevance to those helplines.)

Many trade unions and employers have instituted responsible training programmes about AIDS and HIV infection. The Government has made some efforts too, but appears unwilling to ditch its 'moral majority' supporters, with their 'ban homosexuality' line, in favour of a whole-hearted message about the dangers of certain activities.[24] It has decided that it cannot sidestep the opportunity to have a go at gay men.

Consequently Government persisted in using the language of 'high risk groups' rather than 'high risk behaviours'. Of course in this way it was easy to portray 'male homosexuals' as the highest risk group.

We have passed – almost – the era of treatment being refused to men in road accidents who happened to look effeminate, and who 'therefore' might have AIDS.

The matter of AIDS and HIV infection as an issue in the counselling work of gay helplines is considered in chapter 3.

Parliament

Despite the media presentation of AIDS and HIV infection – or perhaps because of it – parties with manifestoes committed to enshrining gay and lesbian equality in law received over 55 per cent of the vote in the 1987 UK General Election.[25] The electors of the inner London constituency of Islington South and Finsbury re-elected Chris Smith with an increased majority. This was the first time that a publicly acknowledged gay man or lesbian had been elected to the House of Commons.[26] Yet within six months of the election two public events had reversed 25 years of progress made towards gay and lesbian equality.

One was the introduction in December 1987 of clause 28 into the Local Government Bill. Back-benchers David Wilshire and Dame Jill Knight introduced into a bill designed to curb the powers of local authorities a clause which the proposers indicated was designed to reduce the limited rights of gay men and lesbians. The clause sought to prevent local authorities from 'promoting homosexuality'.[27]

The Government declared its support for the clause immediately despite having rubbished a similar proposal only one year before, and the clause was duly passed, though by a much smaller majority than the Government usually commands.

It would appear that this section of the Act (now enacted) will have little effect both because of its loose drafting and because of the alteration of the notion to 'intentional promotion'.[28] However, the public debate surrounding the inclusion of the clause raised the notion of 'homosexual propaganda' and even gay helplines were not immune from some attack.

The Church of England

The other public event which reversed progress occurred at the November 1987 session of the 'parliament' of the Church of England, the General Synod. A motion was passed, by a large majority, which amounted to an all-out attack on gay men and lesbians.

The nature of the debate in the General Synod owed more to mass hysteria than to the careful and caring deliberations of an elected assembly of Christians. Evidence which, it was claimed, fairly represented the lifestyles of gay men was presented by the leaders of a witch-hunt against gay clergy. This evidence was allowed to go unchallenged despite being fundamentally flawed.

The atmosphere of fear and hatred engendered caused many members of the Synod to vote in support of a motion with which they fundamentally disagreed in fear of the consequences of being seen to do otherwise.[29]

The year 1988 has seen further examples of this mass hysteria emanating from the Church of England:

- Several diocesan bishops have declared their intention to sack all gay clergy in their charge, and others have declared that they have none working in their diocese. The role of a diocesan bishop is to be the pastor to the clergy working in his diocese. Any bishop who declares that he has no gay clergy working in his diocese is either such a bad bishop that he knows nothing of the lives and loves of the clergy in his charge, or he is deceiving himself. I note that some bishops (a very few) have recognised the debt which the Church owes to hard-working gay clergy.[30]
- The authorities of the Diocese of London pursued in the appropriate ecclesiastical court, at vast expense, a successful action to remove the Lesbian and Gay Christian Movement from the office in a city church which it had occupied for 12 years. Sadly, the authorities presented material in evidence which was seriously flawed. This left observers wondering why the authorities chose to believe evidence which was, frankly, unbelievable.[31]

British Telecom

One apparently trivial matter which has also had an impact on the context in which gay helplines work concerns British Telecom, the recently-privatised telephone company. In 1986 it decided to permit private chatlines and datelines to operate and to charge a fee. Many chatlines and datelines have been established, including specialist ones for gay men and lesbians.

The existence of datelines may have some long-term impact on the number of personal contact advertisements in gay and lesbian magazines and newspapers, but they are unlikely to have any serious impact on helplines. However chatlines may have an impact. Callers may telephone numbers which are widely advertised in the national, local and gay press and be lined up with whoever is currently chatting on the line.

There is little evidence yet that the existence of these lines has had a marked affect on the numbers of calls made to gay helplines, though it may be that the type of calls has been affected. On the one hand, those who simply want to chat can now do so without telephoning a gay helpline, but on the other hand, those who have serious problems are sometimes referred to their local gay helpline by others on the chatline.

The complete list of gay helplines is very long. It contains the branches of FRIEND, many Lesbian and Gay Switchboards, separate women's only lines, specialist lines for Christians, young people, and other particular groups, and specialist lines for those with legal and parental problems. In addition there are those lines operated from within the gay world specialising in problems concerning AIDS and HIV infection.

Gay helplines in a typical region

So we have seen something of the historical development of gay helplines and something of the social context in which they now have to operate. An outline of a typical region and its gay helplines may help put the focus of this book in context.

No region such as the one described here actually exists, but the description contains elements of many and I hope it will assist readers in reading the rest of this book.

First the geography and demography of the region. The region has a centre with a population of between one and two million living in a conurbation, and it has four sub-centres each with a population of between 150,000 and 400,000. In between these there are many smaller towns and a lot of countryside, so the region has a total population of between four and five million.

In the regional centre there are four gay-related helplines. One of them, the biggest both in terms of number of callers and number of volunteers, is called the Lesbian and Gay Switchboard and has a staff of about 30, about three-quarters of them men. That line sees itself as an information agency, providing the region's gay men and lesbian women with up-to-date information on social venues and on social and political events. It also acts as an accommodation agency, an employment agency, and a focus for advertising new gay-related commercial and social ventures. It is also a feeder service for those specialist helplines it trusts, referring people with particular difficulties which its own volunteers are unable or unwilling to handle themselves.

The second of the helplines in the regional centre is Lesbian Line. It seeks calls from women who see themselves as lesbian and from women who are thinking about the possibility of seeing themselves as lesbian. In the main the volunteers (all women) regard themselves as lesbian feminists and from within that political and ideological position they assist their sisters through whatever difficulties they may be having. The line operates collectively, as a matter of principle, and its counselling style is interventionist in that assistance and guidance are offered where appropriate.

The third of the helplines in the regional centre is called FRIEND, which seeks to be the referral point for those callers with problems and a welfare agency for gay men and lesbians. Callers to the Lesbian and Gay Switchboard will be referred to FRIEND if they present problems more difficult than the volunteer feels able to handle or which seem likely to be more time-consuming than the volunteer feels is appropriate for a helpline which is primarily an information service.

The fourth helpline in the regional centre is an AIDS line, founded in the last three years by some volunteers from other helplines. It sits uneasily in a list of *gay* helplines because it maintains that it serves more than just the gay community in its desire to help people with concerns about AIDS and HIV infection. The majority of its volunteers are gay men or lesbians, or heterosexual people who have a lot of contact with the gay world. It is regarded by the medical profession as being a gay organisation – whatever it may say about itself.

Outside the regional centre, with its four helplines each operating on several evenings each week, are the four smaller centres of population, each of which has had a small helpline at some time in the past. Two of these flourish, one called Lesbian and Gay Switchboard, and the other called FRIEND (the names and the national affiliations reflect history rather than any clear difference in perceived function). The third, called Gayline, has recently restarted after a break. A fourth closed only recently. These three helplines all try to offer a general information and listening service for all men and woman who telephone them. However, since one of them has very few women volunteers, and another has none, there are circumstances where this is very difficult.

In their inability to specialise these three small helplines often try to cover more than their volunteers are able to handle. Whether or not calls are forwarded to their regional specialist gay helplines depends on the nature and extent of any rivalries.

So the mythical region contains seven helplines, each with its own history and its own emphasis.

In London, alongside a helpline which serves essentially as a national helpline referring many of its callers from outside the metropolitan area to regional and local helplines (London Lesbian and Gay Switchboard), there are also small area helplines, not unlike the small helplines in local centres in the typical region.

There are also located in London almost all of the national helplines which specialise in one field of concern, such as legal, medical, parental, religious and several others. Whether or not these specialists receive referrals from local and regional helplines seems to depend on three factors: a helpline's willingness to refer calls to anyone at all; the reputation of the specialist helpline; and the apprehension with which local volunteers view the specialist subject concerned. If it is something with which they feel particularly uncomfortable then they may refer *too* readily.

Balancing influences

Now to the balance which *gay* helplines strike between the pressures and influences upon them. Where do gay helplines stand on the issue of 'evangelising'? Do they express humanitarian concern? How do they balance these influences against pressures of an apparently hostile world and a cosy ghetto?

Humanitarian concern can readily be seen as an influence on the practice of all gay helplines. However, it may not always be clear just how important are the ideals of gay liberationists and feminists.

However a synthesis between humanitarian concern and liberationist ideals seems to have emerged which is tempered (to a greater or a lesser degree) by the realities of the lives of the gay men and lesbians who are the volunteers and by the vibrancy of the local gay world of which they are a part.

Volunteers

It is important that readers do not get the idea that all gay helplines volunteers are fired with gay liberationist zeal, or radical feminist enthusiasm. This notion simply does not stand up.

Volunteers enter the service of helplines, and gay helplines are no exception, for a wide variety of reasons. Frequently this is expressed simply as a desire to help. For each volunteer there is a personal balance between humanitarian concern, a desire to further some set of ideals and a desire to 'help others like me'. There is also a desire to improve their own sense of well-being, perhaps through helping others, perhaps through meeting new people.

Like most gay men and lesbian women, gay helpline volunteers live lives which are a compromise between a cosy gay ghetto and a world which either ignores their gay or lesbian identity or opposes their very existence. The ghetto comprises fellow lesbians and gay men and has its own substructures. Like many gay men and lesbians, volunteers get annoyed at society's failure to accord them equal rights. Like many they feel frustrated that many lesbians and gay men are so ground down by (real or imagined) hostility that they cannot function properly as loving and lovable human beings.

The balance struck between motives is an individual one for each helpline volunteer. The acceptability of particular views among potential volunteers on any helpline is something which each helpline decides for itself.

Like many gay men and lesbians, volunteers are ambivalent about their specialist gay world, a gay ghetto. The desirability of special worlds was considered in general (earlier in this chapter) and questions were posed about it. The parallels to these questions in a gay context are:

- Should there be communities where the common basis is a disposition to sexual attraction to people of the same sex? In other words, should there be gay and lesbian communities (what is called the 'gay world' in this book)?
- Is it any part of the role of a telephone helpline to encourage the development of such communities?

These questions are very difficult to answer. There *are* such communities, and there *is* a gay world. Liberals often claim that if there were no hostility towards gay men and lesbians then there would be no need for a gay world. The radical reply is that if there were no hostility no one would notice whether there was a gay world or not.

Each gay helpline has its own relationship with the gay world; it is of it and yet not in it. It acts as some sort of link between the outside world and the gay world. It has its own balance between all the influences upon it.

Empowerment without exploitation

For the most part, it seems that gay helplines operate within the grey area between evangelising and caring. They seem to take a position which can be described as 'empowerment without exploitation'.

Volunteers in the main seem to try to empower callers to make decisions about their own lives. They do this by helping callers find the courage to believe in themselves and in their abilities to make decisions about their lifestyles, untrammelled by convention and unencumbered by feeling the need to fulfill the expectations of those around them. The following are two examples.

A caller may feel empowered to explain to her aged parents that they cannot assume that merely because she is unmarried, she will *automatically* give up everything to look after them while they have no such expectations of her married siblings. A male caller may feel empowered to reject the wider world's requirements that all men make oppressive remarks against women.

Gay men may feel empowered to stand firm with others against hostility when the gutter press raises anti-gay scares related to AIDS which put people's livelihoods at risk – or to stand firm against those who would hound out of the area a man who was HIV positive, or a woman who reared her children with her woman partner.

That could be thought of as humanitarian concern except when you consider the views of the opponents of gay men and lesbians, through whose eyes this empowerment seems to be an ideological position designed to change society. It must be remembered that gay men and lesbians are in a unique position in society in that their opponents do not recognise their right to exist in the first place. In the debates on the Wilshire/Knight Clause 28 it became clear that many of its proponents, both within and outside Parliament, wished 'homosexuality' to be eradicated entirely from our society. The more liberal of them merely wanted gay men and lesbians to disappear from view.

Such a position, well-known in gay circles, but often forgotten outside, engenders fear in many (and I am sure that this is intended). Helpline volunteers have to contend with this fear in themselves as well as in callers and some do so by withdrawing further into the comparative comfort of a gay ghetto and advance its values and its apparent security. More often volunteers become more concerned to advance gay rights and to ensure that callers are introduced to these issues as soon as possible.

On the other hand volunteers help callers resist when they feel that they are being exploited by the wider world or by the gay world in a variety of ways.

Examples of the exploitation of the wider world are legion. Details of the latest attacks on gay men and lesbians – or at least some of them – can be found in newspapers and magazines designed for a gay and lesbian audience. In late 1988, the largest of these are *Capital Gay* and *The Pink Paper* (weeklies), *Gay Times, Gay Life* and *Gay Scotland* (monthlies). The mainstream press (including the so-called quality papers) rarely print stories concerning attacks on gay men or lesbians, or stories reporting the many successes of gay men and lesbians in their fight for equal rights, unless there can be drawn out of the story an anti-gay line. Demonstrations of 30,000 lesbians and gay men for the annual Lesbian and Gay Pride march in London do not merit even one line in the national press.[32]

Volunteers also help callers resist when they are being exploited by the gay world which beckons, for example: empowering women to stand firm against increased prices in a bar merely because it has decided to permit lesbians to use its facilities; or empowering young men to stand firm in developing their own view of sexual activity with multiple partners, and against being exploited by someone more experienced sexually or more at ease socially who tried to pressurise them into having casual sex. It means ensuring that no one in the gay world takes anyone else for granted.

For many people an acceptable alternative to changing the world is to create a special 'little' world which cushions them from the problems of the 'big' world. Although *finding* that new little world may be a result of being empowered, *staying there* may be a mark of its success in exploiting the feelings of lack of self-esteem of the newly arrived.

Summing up

Each helpline strikes its own balance between the influence on the ways it tackles issues raised by callers and each helpline deals with problems of operation and management in its own way. However the influences on all gay helplines are common and there is a common theme in the consensus each develops round those influences – a consensus described here as 'empowerment without exploitation'. The effect of this consensus is to help callers find the strength to make decisions without feeling oppressed by a hostile world and while feeling the comfort of solidarity with other gay men and lesbians.

It is through a synthesis of influences that gay helplines develop their operating practices, with each helpline making detailed changes in its working practices from time to time, which reflect changes of personnel and changes of social context. Helplines are living social entities, not fossilised institutions.

The next chapters examine in detail what such a synthesis looks like in practice, and how helplines deal with the difficulties that face them every day.

2 Imagine you are a volunteer and the telephone rings

Imagine yourself as a volunteer on a gay helpline. The telephone rings while you are on duty.[1] You answer it with the set form adopted by that particular helpline, perhaps:

'Gay Switchboard, how can we help you?'

How can you help? Can you help at all? The person calling may have struggled for months, even years, to summon up the courage to telephone a service which describes itself as providing help for those with what the caller may consider as 'disgusting feelings', feelings which she or he has been covering up for many years.

From the other end of a telephone how do new callers decide whether the helpline is going to be able to help with the serious problem which faces them?

It is unlikely that such a caller will come to a sudden decision, rather the decision will be taken over a period of time. It may be taken as the call progresses, or perhaps over a series of telephone calls, or it may even take several meetings before the caller decides whether contacting the helpline is of any assistance.

Here we are looking at the start of the process. For some people one way of assessing the helpline may be to see how it deals with silence. Another start to the process is to ask about confidentiality. Quality of counselling and strictness of confidentiality often go hand in hand. However, it is unlikely that a distressed caller will be able to apply rigorous tests to distinguish between the two. Such a caller will be unlikely to be able to analyse the quality of the service offered before discussing his or her own problems.

A third approach may be to shout abuse at the 'filthy perverts' to see how they respond. A fourth, perhaps the most common approach to establishing the value of a helpline is to begin with a trivial question. If a calm voice with a reassuring but businesslike manner answers the question and seems interested in the caller but is not prying, then the caller may be disposed to open up and ask the 'real' question.

Silence – 'What do I say?'

'I had been sitting there on the telephone for 20 minutes, and still nothing, hardly a breath, not even a tap on the receiver. I felt such an idiot, but I kept on making encouraging remarks hoping that something might come of it.'

Every volunteer on every helpline has had experience of finding that there is no one at the other end of the telephone who is prepared to say anything. When the problem is too much to handle the caller may be frightened into total silence. Even finding that the telephone number is actually answered at all may be frightening, because it is a telephone number which claims to help people with the awful 'problem' that has wracked the caller for years.

'No words spoken' constitutes the largest groups of calls received by many helplines. The vast majority of these are calls which are terminated immediately the telephone is answered or where the telephone is found to be dead on lifting the receiver. However some last for a long time. What factors do helplines take into account in deciding how to deal with silence?

There are three types of calls which are superficially similar to the silent call but which require different handling. These are calls from (or to) faulty telephones, calls from people with very serious speech impediments and calls from deliberate time wasters.

Some helplines treat silence as most people treat it on a private telephone: if no speech is heard after an 'ordinary' waiting period then the receiver is replaced. If adopted by a helpline such a policy fails to differentiate between a silent caller and a caller in one of the three superficially similar types.

Means of establishing whether or not there is a fault in the telephone vary depending on the type of equipment. However, one of the advantages of the introduction of advance payment payphones is that the volunteer is no longer left wondering whether the silence merely means that the money mechanism is faulty.

Being tongue-tied is a phenomenon many have experienced at times of apprehension. Occasionally, however, a caller will have a particularly severe speech impediment which, accompanied by feelings of apprehension, may mean that no recognisable words are heard by the volunteer. Such situations require patience: patience which volunteers seem to have in these cases whatever their view of waiting for (actually) silent callers.

Some silent calls may be designed to deliberately waste the time of the helpline in order to abuse the services offered.

Different views of silent callers

One view is that callers are seekers of a service which is available to them through the telephone. The service is available on a 'take it or leave it' basis, the helpline does not seek to impose itself on its callers, nor does it expect to be imposed on unduly by them.

This view is typical of those helplines who see their primary function as a community information resource. If a caller wants a chat, or needs further help, then the agency will attend to the matter but it will not offer such facilities. These information services, therefore, rarely attempt to engage a silent caller in conversation. Beyond a simple statement of what the service exists to provide and, perhaps, suggesting that the caller telephones again, the telephone receiver will be replaced after a short pause if no response is forthcoming.

A rather different view is that 'troubled souls' are seeking rest and consolation, and that the helpline exists to help them in their search. Therefore any hold-up in communicating presents the helpline with a challenge, the challenge to create an environment where callers feel sufficiently at ease to discuss their problems with the volunteer.

Helplines holding this view insist that however verbose or silent the caller, volunteers must never terminate a call. They learn best how to use their voices, their manner, and their words to encourage the caller to communicate – even non-verbally if necessary – *anything* to encourage the silent caller to communicate.

A third view of silent calls, in between the other two, is that some callers will consciously test out what is on offer from the telephone helpline before trying to put into words their requests for assistance. Helplines holding this view see it as essential to portray in the first few minutes as good an image as possible of the helpline and of the services it offers. It is not, thereafter, necessary – and perhaps not even desirable – to sit the caller out, because the caller may feel threatened by excessive talking but may feel unable to replace the telephone receiver until the volunteer has stopped talking.

The silent one talks

In helplines which take the second view or the third view there are instances reported of volunteers sitting it out for over an hour, sometimes with nothing more than the caller's breathing to indicate that there is anybody at the other end. Much more often their experience is that the silent call will last only a couple of minutes.

Then, either the call will finish without anything having been said, or the caller will speak. The silence will have lasted long enough for the volunteer to have said something about what the helpline tries to offer, and long enough for the caller to decide whether to say something.

The response may be anything from an abusive remark to a polite indication that this helpline does not offer what the caller seeks, or the beginning (albeit delayed) of an 'ordinary' call.

There are many occasions when an otherwise silent caller will respond to a request to indicate that they are still there – a cough, or some other noise. The friendliness of the volunteer's voice may reduce the level of threat the caller feels sufficiently for him or her to communicate in some way, but not sufficiently for them to reply verbally.

Tedious though some volunteers find them, systems such as 'one tap on the telephone for yes, two taps for no' sometimes establish communication. Such systems are only of real use in filtering the caller. They can be used to establish whether the caller is male or female, so the volunteer may present details about the helpline and those of its services which seem to be particularly relevant to the caller. In the case of a caller of one sex being spoken to by a volunteer of the other sex, a helpline with volunteers of both sexes may be able to arrange for a volunteer of the same sex as the caller to be brought in on the call. There are many instances where this has induced the caller to speak.

But all this assumes that it is important to persuade the caller to speak. Perhaps volunteers do callers a disservice by attempting to persuade them out of their silence. To know that the service exists and to hear a carefully rehearsed, gentle statement about the work of the helpline may be sufficient on such an occasion. A common sign-off sentence from those helplines who terminate silent calls after a suitable period is: 'We know how difficult it is for some people to speak to us when they first telephone us, but often they phone back later when they are ready to speak, and we are pleased that they do.'

Confidentiality – 'Is anyone listening?'

'This is confidential isn't it? I don't want my mother to know I am phoning you.'

'You don't mind if I call myself John, but you can never be sure who might hear us?'

'The police aren't listening in are they?'

Because for some people what they want to talk about is too horrible to mention, and because those callers may have difficulty in finding the courage to telephone in the first place, many helplines are very concerned to emphasise their confidentiality. Consequently issues around confidentiality play a major role in most training programmes for volunteers.[2] There is a widely held belief among volunteers that callers will not 'open up', that is they will not divulge the 'real nature' of their concerns, unless they can be convinced that the conversation is confidential.

The credibility of a helpline is at stake, as well as its role in filling a gap in the world of the caller. But that credibility needs to be important to volunteers, as well as apparent to callers. If a helpline claims to operate to confidential standards, then it must ensure that it does maintain that confidentiality, and must be seen to do so as well.

Some helplines – though not all – require volunteers on becoming full members to sign an undertaking to maintain confidentiality at all times. (Such an undertaking permits the volunteer, however, to share with other volunteers what has transpired on the telephone. This is seen as necessary so that callers whose calls are causing difficulties may be discussed, and relevant material on a call may be passed to another volunteer to assist that person to deal with a repeat call.)

But how far does confidentiality go? Some helplines require that volunteers keep confidential the fact that they are volunteers. However laudable such a requirement, it raises an important issue concerning the relationship between a helpline and the special communities it seeks to serve.

No helpline can exist without a body of support, either from the community it seeks to serve, or from those who share its ideals of social service, or from society at large. This support is necessary in order that resources are made available to the helpline to continue its work – both of recruits and of money.

If a helpline is to deserve the confidence of its community, and therefore receive necessary support, it must either have a good reputation (locally or nationally), or it must be staffed by people who are known to be trustworthy, sensible and approachable. But how does a new helpline achieve a good reputation – good enough to generate support?

If it has few national links to depend on, or if there is little trust in the community towards services of its type, then it must rely on those of its volunteers who are held in high regard in the community making their involvement with the helpline widely known.

But this is inconsistent with requiring volunteers to keep confidential that they are volunteers. A balance may need to be struck, therefore, between maintaining a sufficiently high profile to ensure that the service is thought to be worth supporting, but low enough so that potential callers are not deterred by a fear of being answered by someone they already know.

I have not taken into account a view of confidentiality prevalent in early gay liberation circles. This view was that confidentiality itself should be rejected because it panders to those who regard 'homosexuality' as unspeakable, by emphasising the secretive nature of a 'disgusting' act. Very few gay helpline volunteers hold such an extreme position, but its influence may sometimes be detected in helpline discussions on confidentiality.

Secrecy

Associated with the requirement for confidentiality is the notion of secrecy. It is worth considering why some people are so concerned about secrecy when it comes to same-sex sexual activity. For some people getting involved emotionally and sexually with others of their own sex seems to be easy – but for other people it seems to take a great deal of courage. Surrounding the issue is often a great deal of fear.

There are many pressures on men and women not to admit to being involved sexually with others of their own sex. These pressures seem to have changed in the last 20 years. For many they are now surmountable, for others they are not. For some (particularly men) there still seems to be a need to maintain anonymity even with their sexual partners. For others secrecy is partial. Perhaps close friends know but not workmates, or workmates know, but not family, or perhaps it is known only to a network of gay friends and not elsewhere, not even to close friends who are not gay. The permutations seem endless.

For other people there is no secrecy at all, but they are a minority. Frequently gay rights campaigners claim that our society could not cope if there were large numbers of people who were open about their (homo)sexuality. Our society would have to change if it were to realise how many gay men and lesbians there are.

In social environments where there are many who have 'come out' it is claimed that there have been changes. Certain local councils, almost all of them London boroughs, where the elected councils have given clear and apparently unambiguous support for gay rights, are given as examples.

During the debates on the Wilshire/Knight clause 28 of the Local Government Act 1988, it became clear that the political far-right believed that some local authorities genuinely supported the sort of changes which lesbian and gay political activists seek. However, the minute progress towards support for gay and lesbian equality, even in those boroughs dubbed 'loony left', indicates that the far-right were mistaken. Many authorities have a long way to go before they accept basic equalities for gay men and lesbians.[3]

Abusive calls

'Go to hell, queer.' 'He was shouting abuse down the telephone without stopping for breath. I'm broad-minded, but the things he proposed for my body and my soul were, to be polite, unusual.' (Richard, volunteer)

Threats, abuse and hoaxes are a normal part of the work of any helpline dealing with controversial or emotionally charged issues.

Within gay helplines there is a widely held view that these come mainly from two groups. The first of these are children who are beginning to question sex and sexuality. They hear views about 'queers' and 'lezzies' from other children, from teachers or from parents, but in order to make up their own minds about such matters they want to hear what one sounds like. So abusive calls from children are not really abusive, they are simply a part of a child's process of building up a picture of sexual orientation for his or her own development. The need to be abusive may be merely a reflection of the education they (fail to) receive through school and family.

The second group is adults who are confused about their own sexuality. The argument runs that the only adults who need to be abusive are those who, consciously or sub-consciously, are running away from their own feelings for people of their own sex. They are the only ones who bother to argue against gay and lesbian rights, or who need to vent their feelings through threats or abuse to a helpline.

Dealing with abuse

How do helplines deal with these types of call? Is the widespread view that abuse calls come from these two sources reasonable, and is it supported by evidence?

If we receive an abusive call on our private telephones, many of us, almost by instinct, will only just avoid being abusive in return, and will terminate the conversation immediately after stating why we are putting the telephone down. Some people argue that helplines should adopt the same policy. What are the arguments for doing more than that?

Those helplines which see themselves primarily as an information resource seem to adopt a particularly defensive posture towards abusive calls. Operating within a sub-culture those helplines reflect its aspirations and fears. Being at the edge of that world, where it connects (as it were) with the rest of society, volunteers feel responsible for defending their world.

Adults who shout abuse down the telephone are often seen as part of a general pattern of attacks on the gay world. The frustration and anger being vented, it is argued, is sometimes followed by physical attacks, either on individuals or on gay-related social facilities, such as pubs, clubs, discos or gay centres. So volunteers will argue back, defending the gay world by quick responses to abuse, in an effort to defuse any violent feelings towards the gay world which the caller feels. An example is 'So some gay men are limp-wristed, but some others are rugby players.'

In helplines where the influence of gay liberation is particularly strong volunteers *appear* to respond in a similar fashion; they seek to defend. However the volunteer's responses are likely to be more forthcoming, more likely to challenge the assumptions underlying the words of abuse used. Questions like, 'So what's wrong with being a queer?' or 'What do you think a queer is then?' directly challenge the caller on the caller's own terms.

The very fact that callers can be bothered – for whatever reason – to contact a gay helpline is seen as an indication that they have some personal interest in same-sex relationships. Directly challenging the caller's abuse, rather than praising the value of variety (for example), seeks to challenge the notions about sexuality and masculinity which underly the abuse.

Many volunteers feel that the best way of handling an abusive adult caller is to recognise the anxiety being demonstrated by the abusive remarks, pay as little attention as possible to the content of the remarks, and pay as much as possible to the emotions.

Some volunteers claim that, in those instances, it helps to distance the helpline from whatever it is that the caller is abusing (same-sex relations in general, usually), by stressing that the helpline exists to help people with problems. By avoiding identifying the helpline with the substance of the abuse, the volunteer can sometimes bring the abuse to a halt. All but the very angry are concerned not to give vent to their feelings to the 'wrong people'.

Responses to children who make abusive telephone calls are more consistent, and more tolerant. Children who find, remember, and then use the telephone number of a gay helpline are likely to be thinking hard about their own sexuality. Some of them may become participants in the gay world in due course or, if not, they are likely to be more tolerant than their peers, particularly if they have been well treated over the telephone.

Perhaps it does not matter whether helplines are correct in their views about the sources of abusive calls since those views are held throughout the field and they are acted on. While it could be claimed that their views on the matter are subjective, they are the nearest which society has to 'experts' on the matter, and it would be very difficult to devise a way of examining the matter further.

Volunteers from a variety of gay helplines have produced anecdotal evidence of people who admit that they made abusive calls either when still teenagers or when they were particularly confused about their sexuality.

Abusive calls do not form an important part of the work of most helplines, though there seem to be two groups of exceptions. One is Lesbian Lines (which have been explicitly excluded from *detailed* consideration in this book) and the second is newly established lines in small communities away from large conurbations.

When a gay helpline opens, abusive calls seem to flood in. It is as if there is a constant amount of abuse for helplines available in every area. Where a helpline has been operating for a long time, this constant amount only feels like a small trickle, but when a new helpline opens it is like breaching the wall of a dam.

So a caller may have gone through any of the stages, being silent, questioning confidentiality or being abusive, before raising the issues which caused her or him to telephone the helpline.

3 What Do Callers Ask?

What do callers ask, and how do volunteers answer their questions? What does the way they answer and the answers they give tell us about the helpline, about the volunteers and about attitudes towards 'homosexuality' in our society? The most important and most frequently raised of the issues brought to the attention of gay helplines are 'Am I gay/lesbian?', 'Will I get AIDS?' and 'Where is the best gay pub in town?'

'Am I gay/lesbian?

This, the most common of all questions to gay helplines, comes in a variety of forms, for example:

'I don't want to be gay – nobody can make me, can they?'
'How do you know you're a lesbian?'
'I don't seem able to make friends with girls. Does that mean I'm queer?' (a 17-year-old man)

Before looking at the question and at answers to it, another example, from 19-year-old Simon, must not be forgotten:

'I saw a programme on television which made out that to have sex with another bloke was some big deal. I have sex with blokes and girls – so what's the fuss about?'

Questions of the 'am I gay/lesbian?' type are usually asked by people who are reaching adulthood, though there are a number of older inquirers, often those who are reassessing their lives after some important event, death of a loved one, or divorce, perhaps. The 'what's the big deal' variant from Simon was rarely heard 10 or 15 years ago. Volunteers often find this type of call very difficult because they are unwilling to take Simon at face value, not because his sentiment is unusual among young gay men and young lesbians, but because if Simon is experiencing no difficulties why is he contacting a helpline?

However, Simon's need to ask the question may mean that he has failed to understand the nature of the repressive attacks of the late 1980s. Therefore many volunteers are wary of mentioning, for example, cases of discrimination against gay men – cases which demonstrate by their frequency that fear of gay lifestyles leads to violence – lest they induce fears in the caller, fears which, in other callers, the volunteer will be trying to diminish.

To 'be' or to 'do'

Theologians, medical researchers and social scientists have debated for over 100 years the issues surrounding the 'Am I gay?' question.[1] In order to see the context in which gay helplines deal with this question it is necessary to summarise some of the arguments advanced.

One view of sexuality is that there are two basic types of people, those who are gay and those who are not. What separates these types is that gay people are fundamentally attracted to people of their own sex, and the others are fundamentally attracted to people of the opposite sex.

In short, gay is something that one is, and therefore it should be possible to find an easy 'yes' or 'no' answer to the question 'Am I gay?'. (Some supporters of this view also hold that there is a third type of person, the bisexual. Others regard such people as merely those who have yet to accept their basic sexual identity.)

Another view of sexuality is that people express their sexuality with others. For some, all the people they express their sexuality with are of their own sex, for others all of the people they express their sexuality with are of the opposite sex; and for yet other people, some are of the same sex and some of the opposite sex. *Sexual activity* can be described – but people cannot be *categorised*.

In short, 'homosexuality' is something that one *does*, and therefore the question 'Am I gay?' cannot be answered in the form asked. Supporters of this view recognise that there are people who do not express their sexuality genitally (for example, those who take a decision to be celibate). Supporters also recognise that there are people who express their sexuality non-genitally without realising that they are expressing their sexuality. Many social psychologists claim that almost everything we do in friendship is an expression in one form or another of sexuality.

To ask why

Cutting across these two views of sexuality are other dimensions. One of these concerns the question 'Why?'. Why are some people gay or lesbian, while others are heterosexual? (Or the question can be put in other ways, for example; why do some men have sex with other men, while others have sex with women?)

Arguments between geneticists, physiologists and psychologists have raged for many decades and have achieved little – except, perhaps, to remind us how easy it is to slip from scientific argument into moral prescription. Extra chromosomes, differences in physique, differences in home environment, and social and family surrounding have all been advanced as possible explanations of why some people are gay or lesbian, or do 'homosexual' acts. Rarely have these debates been couched in neutral terms.[2]

Rarely is it questioned why the idea of causality should be applied at all. It is usually: 'What are the causes of "homosexuality"?' and only occasionally the more neutral 'What causes some people to be gay or lesbian and others to be "heterosexual"?' This lack of neutrality leads to the second dimension which cuts across the be/do debate, the moral dimension.

So the view of some feminists – that to declare her independence from the dominance of men a woman should engage in sexual activity with another woman – is simply beyond the comprehension of those who are seeking causes of 'homosexuality',[3] since it cannot *both* have a cause *and* be a matter of personal choice.

Right or wrong

Are sexual acts between men, or between women, 'right' or 'wrong'? Are they acceptable only when the people concerned cannot have sex with members of the opposite sex? Are they second-best? Or are they better than sexual acts with people of the opposite sex?

In the eyes of much, but certainly not all, of British Christianity and British Jewry, same-sex acts are contrary to the will of God in every possible circumstance, and to condone the commission of such acts in any circumstance is also contrary to the will of God. It is not the province of this book to enter into detailed debate with those who hold this view, nor do I propose to discuss the attitudes of Islam and other world religions.

When the 'contrary to the will of God' argument is advanced it is usually supported by reference to portions of Jewish and Christian scriptures. For reasons contained in a collection of papers edited by the author, scholarly study of the content of some of the portions of scripture usually cited, and of the context and importance of all of them, have rendered these portions inadmissable as evidence in a proper debate on the subject.[4]

Unfortunately for those who seek a re-assessment by the Christian churches of their views on same-sex acts, scholarly study is rarely of use in discussions by opponents of same-sex acts. Careful investigations of translations, meanings and cultural environment are exercises which are viewed with suspicion or hostility.

Those gay men and lesbians who are practising Christians find themselves in the middle of an exchange of hostilities in this matter, between those for whom Jewish and Christian scriptures have no importance and those who claim that these scriptures are of ultimate significance but who refuse to submit the material to scholarly investigation.[5]

Moral pronouncements (whether from the churches or, in the late 1980s, from the government) are of little importance to the vast majority of people in our society. Most people who object to sexual acts between people of the same sex do so as an expression of fear of the unknown and rely on notions such as: 'It is unnatural'; 'It is abnormal'; or simply 'It is wrong'.

Objectors are rarely prepared to be convinced by any rational argument or supporting evidence. So evidence about the large number of societies – or the larger number of animal species – in which same-sex acts occur and seem to be accepted is rarely worth presenting to counter charges of 'unnatural'.[6]

Notions of abnormality are even harder to deal with. I suppose that the idea of a 'normal' 40-year-old man in Britain is: white; married to his only wife; has at least one child by her (and none by any other women); has a car; and is buying a house using a mortgage. But only about one-sixth of 40-year-old men actually meet all these criteria of so-called normality.[7]

Discussions about sin, and about right and wrong, are difficult to conduct. In general people have views which they are unable to justify. These views may come from childhood, from the media, or from people's social surroundings.

Volunteers, particularly those for whom gay liberation ideals are important, often feel very bitter towards the media, believing that much of the media concentrates on the allegedly sordid nature of a few same-sex liaisons without any alternative evidence which would present lesbian or gay relationships in a more favourable light.

How does the volunteer answer?

The question asked of the helpline volunteer, therefore, is a question which involves whether the caller feels personally at ease. It revolves around the ability of the caller to take risks with family and friends and around making decisions which may not be easy to reverse, and, underneath all of these, it revolves around the be/do debate.

The question 'How do I know if I am gay?' receives two sorts of answers. One involves discussing with the caller why it is important to 'know' at all. The caller may be assisted – empowered – by a discussion of the need to find a label for her feelings. It may be that there is no need for a label after the caller has thought again about her feelings of unease about lesbianism. She may be reassured when she considers afresh society's antagonism and feels empowered to stand above it when making decisions about her life and relationships.

But more often than not a caller is not able to deal with this sort of answer. Where a caller needs to pursue the question it is almost universally answered by questions such as 'Which of a couple, a man or a woman, walking down the street together do you automatically look at?', 'Who catches your eye in a crowd?', 'Who do you fancy?' and 'Who are you thinking about when you masturbate?'

The answer to these inquiries is often taken to provide the definite answer to the question. For example, if a man always fantasises about men then he is gay, if he fantasises about women, then he is not. If he fantasises sometimes about men and sometimes about women then he is bisexual.

This may be a useful rule of thumb, but is it an adequate answer to the question? At *one* level it is inadequate since guilt feelings about, or fear of, sexuality may be so great that the caller's 'fantasy mechanism' may be in a mess. So, for example, a man who would fantasise about men is forced by his guilty feelings to fantasise about women. (This argument may be used another way: despite the pressures on their 'fantasy mechanisms', if callers admit that their masturbation fantasies are for their own sex, then there can be no doubt that they are gay.)

Nobody – not least callers – can expect all volunteers working on gay helplines to be conversant with the complexities of current scientific and theological debates surrounding sex between people of the same sex. However, it seems important that each volunteer should be aware of the major strands of debate so that they can decide why they are out of their 'depth' on any particular subject, and can avoid making rash statements.

The desire to help

But there is another level at which the masturbation test, if it may be called that, must be viewed. At this other level it *is* an adequate indicator of an appropriate answer to the 'How do I know if I am gay?' question. But first it is worth examining, in general, how volunteers with a desire to help would be likely to deal with any question.

To deal with callers 'where they are', rather than to try to impose some theory on them, seems best to most volunteers, particularly if the theory seems to remove the caller's freedom of choice. Without some element of choice it is likely to seem pointless to assist callers through their problems. It merely becomes an exercise in persuading the caller to accept the inevitable. So, following this line of argument, volunteers *might* be expected to adopt a 'do' approach to the question, at least in their initial deals with the caller.

But this seems *not* to apply to most responses to the 'Am I gay?' question. Most volunteers consider it easier to help people towards a personal acceptance of their desire for sex with others of their own sex if they can first feel that it is not their 'fault' or 'responsibility' that they have these desires; in other words, if they can first see themselves as 'being' gay.

If callers are horrified by what they think of themselves and their desires, then they will seek ways of altering that situation. There are two obvious ways of doing this. One is by no longer having 'these disgusting desires', and the other is by believing that these desires are not blameworthy because they are predetermined and not subject to the free choice of the caller.

There are many social pressures on callers to believe that sex with others of their own sex is unacceptable. But still they desire these relationships, and those desires are sufficiently strong to overcome their fears of telephoning a gay helpline. Either the pressures are to be ignored, or the desires are to be submerged.

By using the 'be' approach, by thinking of the emotional and spiritual dimensions of identifying with one's own sex, the pressures can be acknowledged and put into some perspective, and the desires can be acknowledged and accepted. Volunteers concerned to empower callers will want them to recognise those feelings as good. The 'be' approach does not permit that since it only allows neutrality between bad and good, but by removing the disapproval from the feelings, they certainly seem much better to the caller.

Answers?

Many volunteers seek a simple objective test for whether the caller 'is gay or not', and do not wish to enter into the be/do debate, or any other debate concerning science or morality.

In the absence of any other test, the masturbation test must suffice. The spectrum developed by Dr Alfred Kinsey and his team in the 1940s is clearly inadequate on several grounds, not least because it refers only to sexual activity to orgasm, which is patently not a useful test for those who have no genital experience with others at all.[8]

The influence of gay liberation steers the volunteer towards the view that anyone who admits to sexual feelings for their own sex must be gay. Influences from within the gay world will reinforce this 'You are gay/lesbian if you feel you are'. Both of these influences will join together at a practical level, so that volunteers often wish to involve anyone who has a desire for same-sex activity in a gay lifestyle within a gay/lesbian community.

Most gay helpline volunteers assume that all, or almost all, of those who ask the question 'Am I gay?' *are* gay, and consequently the volunteer seeks to involve the caller in the gay/lesbian community at a level which seems most appropriate for the caller.

'Will I get AIDS?'

'My mate Alan wants us to have sex, will I get AIDS? Should I let him fuck me? Will it hurt? What does it feel like?' (Patrick, 18).

The calls which present volunteers with the greatest difficulty of all are those concerned with Acquired Immune Deficiency Syndrome (AIDS) and Human Immuno-deficiency Virus (HIV). There seem to be many reasons for this:

- Most helplines did not have to cope with death or serious illness until AIDS and HIV infection became important.
- While the issue of AIDS and HIV infection is in the public eye, it is seriously affecting the ways in which gay men (and lesbians, perhaps surprisingly) are viewed. It may have had the effect of lowering the number of young callers

40 HOW CAN WE HELP YOU?

investigating the possibility of joining the gay world.
- Gay male volunteers feel some of the disquiet for their own personal health which has swept through the gay male circles.

The dramatic differences between the number of reported cases of people (diagnosed) with AIDS across the country is reflected in the approach of helplines.[9] Those helplines operating in London (and one or two other major cities with high prevalence rates) have had to adjust to deaths among their own volunteers, and among the friends of volunteers, whereas helpline volunteers operating elsewhere may have yet to come in contact with persons diagnosed, and may know personally few, if any, who are aware of being infected with HIV.

What is AIDS?

Acquired Immune Deficiency Syndrome (AIDS) is a new phenomenon of the 1980s. Like other apparently new medical conditions, and like other conditions which cause widespread public alarm, researchers are making new discoveries about it frequently. Any statement about AIDS made in a published volume is likely to be out of date before that book reaches the shelves of the bookshops.[10] Readers seeking up-to-date information should refer to the Terrence Higgins Trust, or to one of the specialist AIDS helplines set up over the last four years. The Terrence Higgins Trust has maintained a steady flow of pamphlets and leaflets which have had considerable impact in diminishing fear within the gay male community, and have also alerted gay men to ways in which they may improve their own health and reduce their chances of becoming HIV antibody positive with the attendant risk of contracting AIDS or an AIDS-related condition.

It is clear now that AIDS is caused by a virus, the Human Immuno-deficiency Virus. For the virus to pass between two people requires intimate contact. Infected body fluid – blood, semen or cervical lubricants – must enter the body of someone else. This occurs most commonly in anal or vaginal sexual intercourse. (Other forms of sex carry much lower risks.) The virus may also pass through infected blood being transfused, or through the use of unsterilised needles used for intravenous injections.

While anal intercourse has always found favour with some mixed-sex couples, it is a sexual style suited more to gay men. And while some people who have sex with members of the opposite sex do have many sexual partners, the situation with gay men has traditionally been different. Until the mid-1980s many gay men had large numbers of sex partners.[11] Social taboos against 'promiscuity' were not present. There was no fear of unwanted pregnancy to dampen enthusiasm for recreational sex. There was a social taboo on having gay sex at all, but break that taboo and where do you stop?

It was into this setting that Human Immuno-deficiency Virus appeared. The response of the body seems to vary, but most often the virus may lie resting for many years (perhaps even for ever) – so allowing it to be passed on unknowingly very widely. For some people illness may appear in a mild form, at least at first, for others death may come more quickly – in months in some cases – after conditions which steadily weaken the body's resistance to infection. The virus is no respector of persons. Death comes quickly to some who are fit and some who are unfit, to some who have a lot of recreational sex and some who have little or none. However, it has become clear that people with AIDS may live a (comparatively) long and fulfilled life through adopting lifestyles (diet, exercise, etc.) and life-attitudes which are positive.

AIDS and helplines

Helplines can only train volunteers to carry out a limited number of tasks. It is unreasonable to expect that a general purpose gay helpline will be able to provide its volunteers with sufficient information on AIDS and HIV infection to do more than reduce the level of anxiety in the caller in terms outlined in this section.

It is, of course, vital that volunteers know, for example, the difference between a diagnosed case of AIDS and a positive test for HIV antibodies. There is still a need for counselling for those who are taking antibody tests, both before the test is taken, and when the result becomes available.

For the most part, it seems a good idea that specialist helplines have come into being to deal with more detailed questions on AIDS and HIV infection. (However the matter of the government-sponsored national AIDSLINES, that poached for a decent hourly wage many volunteers trained by voluntary, poorly-funded, generalist gay helplines is something which caused bitterness and resentment. It also raises important issues about the relationship between this government and the voluntary sector which it claims to support.)

In general terms volunteers on gay helplines have the task of trying to damp individual fears about AIDS and HIV infection while ensuring that the gay community continues to take the issue seriously. The (relatively) considerable improvement there has been (since mid 1987) in the rate of new reported instances of gay men becoming infected with HIV is due in no small part to the efforts of specialist, gay-related agencies and gay helplines working within the gay male community to ensure that as much as possible is known by as many people as possible.[12]

However, the panic about AIDS and HIV infection which seemed to grip part of the gay male community, at its base, concerned lack of self-worth.[13] It concerned the remnants of the feelings which, to some extent, every gay man and lesbian knows: 'What I am is wrong, whatever I do will be wrong'. (Similar feelings are expressed by some black persons in a white society, and some women in a male world.)

Introducing callers to the gay world will usually be insufficient to redress these feelings of negative self-worth; it may need more than merely introducing them. Volunteers have to empower callers. They have to build up their self-image with them. It would seem that only through assisting gay men to come to a new awareness of their positive identity as gay men can the feelings of fear, even panic, and lack of self-worth be dispelled. Empowerment, through learning about gay liberation, becomes all important at a time of group crisis. Even volunteers have had to be reminded of their own worth during the AIDS crisis.

Fears which even the most dedicated male volunteers may have had concerning their own sexual practices and HIV infection had to be tackled through discussion so that the fears were conquered. This included discussions of the meaning of 'safer' sex – and by implication 'least safe' and 'safest' sex. It became clear that without successfully retraining gay male volunteers, successful efforts to help all gay men would be even more difficult.

Mass panic is too strong an emotion to be handled only by calm reassurance by and to a few. The effects of reassurance given over the telephone would have been lost as soon as the caller socialised again unless helplines, and their associated specialist Aidslines, had not tackled the problem head-on.

Most helplines became involved, directly or indirectly, in ensuring that as much useful information as possible was made available to gay men in their catchment areas through leafletting pubs, clubs and organised groups. Without this change of emphasis from the individual to the group activity, a helpline faced with panic among the gay men in its area would have found that same panic enveloping its volunteers.

Two tasks remain for volunteers in addition to dampening fears while ensuring that AIDS continues to be taken seriously. These concern persons infected with HIV, and persons (diagnosed) with AIDS. Body Positive people (as those who know themselves to be infected with HIV are known) need to work through issues concerning who to tell and how; in particular whether, when and how to tell a lover; and whether, when and how to tell a potential lover.[14] The other task is to ensure that practical support is given to all those with AIDS and their friends and families.

AIDS and the future

It is impossible to assess the long-term effect of AIDS and HIV infection on same-sex relations. One possibility is that fewer and fewer people (particularly men) will want to associate themselves with 'being gay', forcing the gay world further underground and setting back all the advances in public perception of gay men and lesbians made in the last 20 years.

Another possibility is that gay men will achieve some sort of consensus on the nature of the gay sexual morality which involves caring for the good health of the other as well as for one's own good health.

Another is that public hysteria will be used to introduce repressive legislation against gay men far beyond anything contained in the Wilshire/Knight section 28.

Another is that the general public will realise that gay men (and their lesbian friends) have done such a good job in educating themselves about AIDS and HIV infection that gay men and lesbians will come to be seen as valuable sections of society. (The evidence for this educational success being that diagnosis rates have increased more slowly than predicted by eminent epidemiologists.) I wonder which it will be.

Sexual techniques

Alongside qustions on AIDS often come detailed questions concerning sexual activity and technique. The detailed questions often come after questions about matters which the caller appears to regard as easier. They have always caused some volunteers problems because the questions often are at a level which some find embarrassing, as does the caller. That in itself says two things about how sex is viewed in our society.

Firstly, it says that many people lack what they regard as vital information about sexual acts, information which they need to obtain from a helpline rather than from friends, books or general conversation. Secondly it says that many people are sufficiently embarassed about the subject of sexual acts that, even with assurances of confidentiality, they need to ask easy questions of a helpline before they get round to this issue.

There is a great deal of ambivalence about sex. Sexual acts are placed on a pedestal, and yet they are widely thought to be, somehow, dirty – and this ambivalence seems to apply both to gay sex and straight sex.

There seems to be an obsessive interest, on the part of some men who insist that they are not gay, in what two men, or more often two women, do as part of their sexual activity. This voyeurism annoys many helpline volunteers, and many helplines insist, for example, that details of what two women 'do in bed' are only discussed (when requested) with women callers, and by women volunteers.

When volunteers are answering questions about sexual techniques they have to explain the range and variety of ways in which people make love or have sex. The joys and dangers of having anal sex need to be explained to Patrick (mentioned on page 39) in a language he understands, which is more likely to be the language of the street than the language of the human biology textbook. The explanations have to be given slowly and graphically and in a manner which does not frighten him unnecessarily.

Are you passive or active?

For many volunteers the most difficult part of a discussion about sexual techniques (once the initial embarrassment has been overcome) is to help callers allow themselves to think about sexual activity more broadly than in terms of sex roles.

To some extent this has become less important since helplines were founded, but there is still presented, from time to time, a desire to find a 'butch' or 'femme' partner, an 'active' or 'passive' partner. The apparent need to ape heterosexual gender roles, or to have roles which can be presented as analogous to old-style heterosexual ones, has also become less important.

This change may be related to three social changes, which may themselves be connected. The first is the slow weakening of gender roles. Women have more opportunity, whether or not they have children, to adopt roles other than 'motherhood' and 'housecraft'. Women's liberationists may regard the changes as insufficient and partial, but they are marked.

The second social change is the openness of some gay men and lesbian women. It is no longer necessary for a same-sex couple who are 'out' to be a pseudo-man and a pseudo-woman. They can now be a couple of men or a couple of women, without any necessary public pretence to be anything else.

The third social change is associated with AIDS and HIV infection. The advent of 'safer sex' guidelines has brought to the attention of many gay men something which many lesbians have always known – that we all have a vast range of sexual activities available to us. Furthermore, the emphases in the 'safer sex' literature on the dangers associated with anal intercourse and with orgasm has led many men to recognise that sex, to be fulfilling, need not necessarily be tied closely to orgasm with its attendant notions of dominance and achievement.

A smoke screen

Occasionally, it would seem, questions about sexual techniques are used as a cover to avoid taking the risks involved in trying to find a sexual relationship. Patrick may be using his fear of anal sex, or his fear of becoming infected with the HIV virus, as a way of avoiding being in a relationship with Alan. The volunteer must ensure that this issue is not hidden behind his request for an explanation of every detail of anal sex.

'Where is the best gay pub in town?'

The seemingly harmless, simple request for information comes in all shapes and sizes. But is it more than it seems? Can the caller really only be telephoning for that?

For gay helplines, the best-known, apparently simple request for information often sounds like: 'Where is the best gay pub in town?'

The volunteer is faced with two problems concerning the question: firstly, is this the real question? Is it all the caller wanted to ask? Is there something underneath this simple inquiry which is troubling the caller? Secondly, if we treat it at face-value, how far should a helpline go in recommending individual commercial enterprises? In this case, should any particular pub have the helpline's 'seal of approval' placed on it?

Giving the caller the information

Some helplines are geared primarily towards the giving of information. For volunteers to withhold information would offend against the underlying philosophy of the helpline, and the volunteer might simply not consider withholding any available information. Callers' requests are treated for what they seem to be, requests for information.

Other helplines, however, adopt a rather different approach. They refuse to give any informtion at all, limiting themselves to a counselling or befriending role, and referring to other helplines any requests for information. Thus they avoid altogether the problems (including the problem of deciding what is and what is not a gay pub for inclusion on some list to be read to all callers).

In the middle are those helplines which seek to help the caller work up to what is the real problem that they want to discuss, allowing any information to be used as an opening gambit, while recognising that some people actually want to know what is, in the judgement of the helpline volunteer, the best gay pub in town.

Volunteers are accustomed to apparently simple information calls which continue: 'by the way, while I'm talking to you, what do you think of . . .?'

One aspect of training for new volunteers is often to help them create easy entry points for the 'by the way . . .' calls, and a manner which encourages the caller to raise them.

One way to encourage a caller to open up is to deal with the information request in a conversational fashion. A direct answer to information requests provides few entry points, whereas an answer which requires the caller to express preferences, to think about her or himself aloud before obtaining an answer to the request for information, is thought to provide more entries.

So, for example, with the information request about pubs, questions which have been found useful include:

- 'Do you like quiet pubs or noisy ones?' indicates that there is more than one gay pub, and that there is variety within the gay world.
- 'Do you normally go to a pub on your own?' allows a caller who has recently split up with a lover to say 'Until recently I would not but now . . .'
- Giving the opening and closing hours of pubs and clubs allows a caller to say 'I can't stay out that late, my mother would want to know where I was' or 'I can only get away during the lunch-hour, otherwise my husband will find out.'

So the volunteer will be able to make conversation about the mother or the husband or about the caller's knowledge of gay-related facilities, without appearing to pry.

Some of the problems facing those helplines which operate a 24-hour service are different, since any caller may be at a moment of crisis when they are telephoning. This is not the case for most helplines because they operate for only limited periods each week (perhaps two or three hours in the evening or anything from one evening per week upwards), so callers need to plan to telephone. It is the experience of gay helplines that many callers keep the number in their memory for a long period before telephoning, and many of these are mulling over ways in which they may have conversation about a subject which embodies their personal fears.

(One gay helpline – London Lesbian & Gay Switchboard – is the exception to the general observation that *gay* helplines do not offer an immediate service. That switchboard proudly claims to operate throughout the day and night and throughout the year, and is much respected for it.)

The dangers

But there is a danger. Callers who are pushed too hard may be frightened off altogether, put the telephone down and never call back. It is possible – indeed it often appears to be the case – that the caller really does want information only. There can be no foolproof test for this. We all have some problems, and (given the right circumstances) we are willing to talk about them.

Some helplines insist that volunteers ask a question like 'what gay pubs have you been in before?' which seems to establish something of a caller's awareness of the gay world before giving out any information. This is designed to prevent the volunteer landing raw new young people into gay pubs without any prior consideration, or to avoid a plea for support from an older inexperienced caller going undetected. It is still important in some cases to ask such a question in order to reduce the chances of giving out information to those hostile to gay men and lesbians.

At the extreme, of course, the caller who is simply seeking information may invent a problem in order to satisfy a volunteer who is determined that the caller must have a problem, and in order to obtain the information sought, which is otherwise being refused. Too much of that and a helpline acquires a reputation for being prying and unhelpful, a reputation which is often difficult to throw off.

Which pub?

Endorsement of individual commercial ventures, and advertising the services of professionals, forms part of the day-to-day work of many gay helplines in the United States.[15] Endorsement and advertising play an extremely important part in the funding arrangement for some of them. A gay bar may negotiate with a helpline to provide a certain level of funding in return for always mentioning (and never unfavourably) that particular bar when information on gay bars is sought by a caller. A lawyer or a doctor may negotiate funding in return for providing those seeking such services with the name concerned.

North American society is geared even more than the UK to the business ethic and competition. Little there is left untouched by capitalism, not even humanitarian ventures. Those devoted to ideals of voluntary service may be saddened that helplines are prepared to accept arrangements for such sponsorship or endorsement even through financial necessity.

The development in North America of Lambda Business Councils and Gay and Lesbian Professional Caucuses may alleviate this situation somewhat, while also providing a useful service to gay men and lesbian women. Lambda[16] Business Councils are specialist chambers of commerce for gay-related business operators. In many large cities in the USA and Canada, the Lambda Business Council is recognised by the general business community as representing a sectional interest, and it has affiliated to its city's chamber of commerce.

Gay and Lesbian Professional Caucuses bring together accountants, lawyers, doctors and others into a specialist gay and lesbian version of Rotarians, Soroptomists or Lions. These caucuses provide an environment where people may have social and intellectual involvement at a point where their personal and professional lives come together.

Lambda Business Councils and Gay and Lesbian Professional Caucuses have proved to be the means by which helplines have escaped from the clutches of raw commercialism. In several cities these organisations have negotiated a funding arrangement with a helpline in return for general promotion of the interests of the members of the organisation.

So the individual volunteer is left with the decision about which, if any, commercial ventures or professional services to recommend if a recommendation is sought. It keeps the forces of capitalism out of the relationship between caller and volunteer and allows the relationship to remain that between two human beings. It serves to encourage gay and lesbian-related businesses and gay and lesbian professionals to join the relevant organisation in order to gain the general benefits of being promoted through the helpline.

Helplines operating in regional centres in North America work in a very different environment to their equivalents in the UK. Two ways in which the environment differ are important here:

- there are much larger, more self-assured and self-identified gay and lesbian 'sub-cultures' in regional centres in North America than in this country
- many more people do a lot of travelling from place to place

Together these two factors mean that there is a greater need for information, and perhaps less need for counselling and befriending.

Outside London there would appear to be insufficient demand for separate Lambda Business Councils because there are too few gay-related businesses.[17] Several professions have established Gay and Lesbian Professional Caucuses, but almost without exception these operate from, or only in, London. Furthermore, attitudes towards 'good works' in this country are more positive and less commercial than in North America. But that still leaves the problem for the helpline and volunteer about whether to recommend a particular gay pub or other venue or enterprise.

Most helplines have tried to avoid being caught in the commercial trap and adopt one of two solutions to the problem. Either the individual volunteers are left to give reasoned answers based on their own judgement of the venues and of the needs of the caller, or, as a matter of policy, a list of all venues is given out so that the caller can make a decision without benefit of the judgement of the helpline or the volunteer.

4 Being a Volunteer

What is it like to be a volunteer? What are the general problems of being a volunteer on a helpline, and particularly on a gay helpline? What general questions is it necessary for volunteers to ask themselves about their work, whatever sort of helpline they are working for?

'Am I good enough to be a volunteer?', 'Should I tell people what to do?' and 'Can I answer anybody or only people like me?' are the most important of these general questions.

Selection and training of volunteers

'Where will we find more volunteers?' is a cry heard from many helplines, whereas others are overwhelmed by applicants. How do people become volunteers on a helpline? How do helplines decide who they want as volunteers?

The criteria for the selection of volunteers which have emerged in over a third of a century of the existence of helplines in the UK contain several common items, whatever the focus of the work of the helpline.[1] These include self-knowledge, compassion, unshockability, adaptability, ability to keep confidences and a sense of humour.[2] Other items include commitment, time-keeping, willingness to place responsibility to callers above all other reasonable considerations, particularly when on duty.

Acceptance of leadership may also be a requirement, though some helplines, as an article of faith, operate on a collective principle, and most – even where power of discipline is vested in a leader – insist on collective decisions about general policy. Given the differences in emphasis apparent between helplines, it is clear that an acceptance of the general philosophy under which the helpline is operating is also essential. Knowledge of the field may also be required. Keeping up to date with new information as it arrives, and ensuring that all volunteers feel at ease in the social environments where they might be expected to introduce callers may also be part of the volunteer's job.

I want to consider these matters by looking at selection procedures and training programmes which are used in helplines currently operating.

Volunteers and training

There is a wide range of types of training programmes mounted for recruits to helplines. Each helpline decides what training programme volunteers must pass through before being 'let loose' on the public by being permitted to answer a helpline telephone.

Not included in my definition of helplines are the open telephone lines (the chatlines) run for profit, where there is no distinction between caller and volunteer since all are the same. These lines merely permit callers to speak to one another and are (it is argued by their supporters) simply an extension of over-the-fence chat with the neighbour. They are not helplines in the sense in which it is used here, though telephoning them may help some people.[3]

Also not the concern of this book are the charlatans: enterprises claiming to be helplines run by people with unacceptable ulterior motives seeking to prey on the troubled and worried. Any *bona fide* helpline, whatever the area of its specialism, is determined to distance itself from the (very few) charlatans.

However, among *bona fide* helplines there is a wide range of methods of training. At one end there are still some helplines with no coherent training programme at all for volunteers. In most of these cases the ruling argument is the small size of the volunteer group: there are so few volunteers that running a formal training programme is deemed to be nonsensical.

For those helplines with only a turnover of one or two volunteers per year, mounting a coherent *group* training programme is indeed nonsensical, but this does not absolve the helpline from devising a coherent training programme for each new recruit.

It would seem that the stream of thinking against any training at all that prevailed in some helplines in the 1960s and the 1970s has almost completely died out. It was argued that all training was irrelevant because being 'good on the telephone' was a gift you either possessed or you did not.

It is worthwhile to examine two different types of training programme offered in large general helplines in provincial centres. There are many variations on both these types, but these are presented to give some indication of the real training which well-organised helplines provide and in order to highlight the strengths and weaknesses of each programme.

Two helplines and their training

Helpline A

Twice a year helpline A announces as widely as it can – by advertising in the gay press, by posters placed in gay clubs and pubs, by word of mouth and through the local volunteer bureau – that new volunteers are being sought. A day is set, usually a Saturday, and all are welcome to present themselves at 9.30 am for a day of discussion of the work of the helpline.

On one of these Saturdays, ten to twelve people present themselves. Many of them are known to one or more of the existing volunteers. Some of these have been actively encouraged to come along. There are a few complete strangers. Almost half of the volunteer team of between 25 and 30 are also present.

The day starts with familiarising exercises (on some occasions it begins with a formal introduction). Then slowly the range of work of the helpline – the types of calls and the problems – is explained and questions sought and discussion encouraged. There are lots of breaks and in the middle of the day lunch is served. The breaks and the meal provide occasions for existing volunteers and potential recruits to talk to one another in a relaxed atmosphere.

The afternoon session concentrates on role playing. Pretending to answer calls, and even pretending to make calls which are answered by others, gives the recruits a foretaste of work on the helpline, and listening to their performance allows existing volunteers to assess the suitability of each recruit. At the end of the day those who wish to do so are invited to apply for admission as a volunteer.

In due course a small group of volunteers interview each applicant and decide whether or not to admit them. In coming to its decision the small group is aware of the reaction of volunteers to each recruit on the open day.

Admission to the helpline as a volunteer may be unconditional and immediate, or a recruit may be attached to a named volunteer for a specified period of (say) three months. The recruit moves on to the telephones from a 'sit by and listen in' position when both recruit and named volunteer are happy about that transfer.

Helpline B

Helpline B runs three training programmes each year, each lasting for six months. Like Helpline A, it advertises itself as widely as possible, but does not specify times for starts of courses, so it receives a steady trickle of enquiries throughout the year. In September, January and April it gathers together all those who have indicated interest in becoming volunteers since the beginning of the last training programme and a small group of volunteers, usually two women and two men, interview each applicant.

Before that interview each enquirer will have completed an application form and will have been given a copy of the helpline's most recent annual report.

Each applicant will have provided the names of two referees, one gay or lesbian and one not, whose opinions on the character of the applicant will be available to the interviewers. As a result of the preliminary interview an applicant may be admitted to the training programme, put on a waiting list, or rejected altogether.

In common with Helpline A, those rejected are informed of their rejection in a positive manner, for example by suggesting that their talents could be used to best advantage in other ways which would benefit the helpline. They may have useful secretarial or fund-raising skills, or they may be skilled in practical tasks concerning the upkeep of the helpline's premises.

Then the training programme begins. It is organised by a team of four volunteers (not the interviewers) and consists of 10 evening sessions. The first six of these sessions, held weekly, cover the material covered in the day session run by Helpline A, but at greater length.

After these six sessions each recruit (except for the occasional one who is thought to be wholly unsuitable) is linked up with another volunteer and sits with that person during his or her next three duty periods. The recruit sees at first hand the work of the helpline, without participating in it directly. Another volunteer gets to know the recruit in addition to the members of the training team and members of the interview panel. Each recruit also meets those who are on duty with his or her link.

The recruit sees the relevance of the role-play work undertaken in the weekly training sessions, including work done 'being the caller' and 'being the volunteer' on a mock telephone system which the helpline has developed.

Session seven of the training programme allows for reflections on the experience of sitting beside the link, and prepares the recruit for listening in on the dumb receiver associated with each incoming line on another three duty periods with their link person.

Session eight allows for discussion of experiences at this stage, and prepares recruits to act as the volunteer, as does session nine. For the six duty periods between session eight and session ten recruits will answer the helpline, with the link volunteer listening on the dumb receiver, ready to take over if the call seems to be going disastrously awry.

The tenth and final session includes a final interview with a new panel who have reports available from the link volunteer and from the training team. So, of a group of, say, 30 volunteers, at least 13 of them – two four-person interview panels, a training team of four and a link volunteer – have some knowledge of the recruit before admission to full membership of the helpline.

Who is accepted?

All sorts of people are accepted as members of helplines, and it seems that the type of training programme does not affect that. Both training programmes find that of those who present themselves initially as recruits, between one-third and one-half are finally accepted as volunteers, a range which is similar to that of the Samaritans.[4] For both training programmes the vast majority of 'drop-outs' are those who decide that they are not suited to the work, or are insufficiently committed to it; outright rejections by the helpline are rare.

The average length of stay of a new full member is about three years in both cases. While both helplines outlined offer a full range of services, from information to befriending and counselling, Helpline A concentrates on information and Helpline B on other aspects of the work.

On-going training

Rudimentary programmes of training for serving volunteers exist in both these helplines. However, most of the on-going training is carried out by means of meetings of volunteers to discuss the business of the helpline, at which difficult calls are discussed, the discussion in itself acting as a form of ongoing training.

Both of these helplines organise occasionally a day away together for the volunteers (maybe once or twice a year). These days provide occasions which are part social and part on-going training, and which serve to enhance group morale.

Part of the on-going training provided for volunteers consists of attending conferences organised by federations of helplines. Such occasions fulfil another important function in that they allow some form of consensus to emerge on ways of operation.

Within FRIEND there have been several attempts since its foundation in 1971 to move beyond the creation of a consensus and create a set of national standards mandatory on all constituent groups. Each of these attempts has met with one major difficulty – resistance to any move towards a strong central structure. Alongside this there has been resistance to any standardisation of the principles upon which these helplines operate. However, despite difficulties in producing *formal* agreement, a high degree of *informal* agreement has always existed about the general ethos of the helplines in the FRIEND confederation.

Sufficient agreement over the aims of the central structure, National FRIEND, has been achieved to allow it to submit an acceptable constitution to the Charity Commissioners and registered charity status was obtained in 1986 for National FRIEND Ltd, a company limited by guarantee.[5] Several of the individual helplines in the confederation have also achieved registered charity status, but each has had to seek it separately.

The degree of informal and formal agreement extends to a programme for establishing new helplines which seems to have stood the test of time, a several times revised guide for volunteers in FRIEND helplines and a programme of monitoring the work of individual helplines operated by the National Committee.

A twice-yearly conference provides an important opportunity for in-service training of befrienders (as volunteers on FRIEND helplines are known), as well as an opportunity for informal consensus on individual topics to be negotiated.

A similar network for lesbian and gay switchboards was formed in 1978.[6] Unlike FRIEND, however, there is one very large lesbian and gay switchboard and a number of much smaller ones. The practices and styles of the large one have been passed on to others by a process of osmosis.

London Lesbian and Gay Switchboard has a high profile, and its apparent success in the eyes of many switchboard volunteers up and down the country has allowed its styles and practices to become a standard against which smaller switchboards may measure their own.[7] The degree of conformity must not be overstated, though it may be seen to have grown considerably over the last decade and more.

The network of lesbian and gay switchboards went into abeyance in 1985. However various regional groupings of helplines run regular conferences for volunteers and these conferences fulfil many functions similar to FRIEND conferences.

The third national link is that of lines run and staffed solely by lesbian women, Lesbian Lines. Volunteers maintain contact with each other through week-end events which allow for experience to be shared between them. Sometimes such events include women volunteers working on mixed (male and female) helplines as well as those who work on women-only lines. Those who attend these events attest to their value and in particular their usefulness in allowing those women who work on helplines where they are greatly outnumbered by men volunteers to benefit from contacts with other women working in similar conditions.

Matching volunteers with the services offered

One of the most difficult tasks in the running of a helpline, and in ensuring that it has the public image it wants with its (potential) client group, is getting the right balance of volunteers – both the right numbers and the right quality.

Without enough volunteers the existing ones will leave because there is so much work that they cannot cope, or, if they stay, the quality of their work will decline through resentment about being overworked. With an excess of volunteers many will get bored and leave because they do not want to sit through a duty period twiddling their thumbs. They may also leave because they are not rostered for enough duties.

Part of the skill of managing a helpline seems to be to judge the amount and variety of telephone service offered and to balance it with the numbers of volunteers – their needs, strengths and weaknesses. Too much service and not enough volunteers leads to poor quality offered by ill-suited, poorly trained and overworked people; too little service and too many volunteers leads to boredom and frustration.

Helplines often find the decision to reduce the service offered heartrendingly difficult to take. It is seen as a mark of failure. Good rational arguments are often used to avoid the need to take the decision. The best of these arguments is that potential callers often note the telephone number and duty times and retain that information hoping to find the courage to call sometime in the future. To find that the number no longer works, or that the helpline is no longer operating at the times noted, is thought to be a major deterrent to callers who have considerable difficulties.

It is argued that it is much easier for a hard-pressed helpline to withdraw from running a support group for callers whom a helpline has encouraged to meet together because of common interest and to whom the helpline offers continuing support. This is because the support group can be urged to continue meeting if it so desires, without helpline volunteers being present at meetings.

Increasing the telephone service offered is much easier – unless the service operates each evening for a substantial period already. Moving into weekday daytime periods requires a great deal of planning and a substantial number of volunteers with free time available at those periods. Widening the service offered, in ways which may also improve the social life of the volunteer team, is more likely to be successful in maintaining and developing morale.

Money comes into this management equation also; there seems to be a relationship between the number of callers and the amount and variety of advertising. It is not just the number of hours for which the helpline operates which matters, it is the amount and variety of advertising of the service which affects the number of callers.

Almost without exception, advertising costs money. Free listings in commercial newspapers and directories and the Public Service Announcements scheme run by some Independent Television stations provide a much needed fillip to the advertising of those helplines which are financially hard-pressed. (Gay helplines often find that free newspapers refuse to include them in listings, and the Public Service Announcements scheme is only open to gay helplines on terms which many helplines regard as insultingly restrictive.)

The management of a helpline, then, needs to balance money-raising for advertising with the extent and variety of the service offered and with the numbers and strengths of volunteers available.

Who calls?

The types of callers depend on the sort of area in which the helpline is situated, the nature of its culture and the attitudes taken to the issue of primary concern to that helpline.

So for gay helplines the type of caller is affected by the image by which its gay and lesbian social environments – pubs and clubs – are known to the general public. It is also affected by the degree of expressed hostility to gay men and lesbians in the area and how much that hostility is expressed in the local media. These matters are general and may only be changed through concerted effort, perhaps by the communities of gay men and lesbian women acting together.

There is, however, one matter the helpline can control which affects the types of caller – advertising. The types of callers depend on the sort of advertising done for the helpline. Let me compare two more helplines, C and D.

Helpline C advertises solely in the local evening newspaper. A small advertisement appears regularly in the 'personal' column without any editorial material or any particular attention being drawn to it.

The other, Helpline D, advertises in a regular newsheet available only to a specialist audience, namely in gay pubs, clubs and organisations and in other venues where there are likely to be a lot of lesbains or gay men. Its advertisements are often prominent and are occasionally supported by editorial material.

Helpline C has a steady flow of callers. Those callers have a broad range of ages and only a small proportion of them raise problems concerning a current gay relationship. Helpline D has an erratic flow of callers, related to the extent and nature of the editorial support, and to the prominence given to its advertisement in the most recent issue of the newsheet.

Helpline D finds itself dealing with problems related to the gay world, its facilities, and to gay relationships to a much larger extent than C. Only rarely does it deal with lonely isolated people who think that they are the only lesbian woman or gay man.

For a short while Helpline C mounted a concerted advertising campaign in a regional teenagers' magazine. This had the effect of shifting the balance of its callers towards that age group, as expected. The helpline considered in advance the likely impact of that advertising and considered what sort of specialist provision for teenage callers it needed to offer and what additional training needed to be provided for the volunteers.

So managing a helpline involves remembering that differing sorts of advertising attracts different sorts of callers. The sort of advertising, of course, has a bearing on the training given to volunteers, it also has a bearing on the reputation of the helpline within its local community.

Because Helpline D advertises in a specialist newsheet, more of its local (in this case gay) community remember its existence. (Many callers choose to forget that they ever called a helpline after they have become integrated into a gay-related social environment for a few years. Reasons for this are difficult to assess, but perhaps it is not socially acceptable to have needed to call a gay helpline to gain access to the gay world. Perhaps one ought to have been sufficiently mature, or sufficiently streetwise, to have found that world without needing the help of a telephone helpline.)

'Should I tell people what to do?'

'Jane kept on asking me what she should do. I didn't want to tell her, because I am not in her shoes.' (Margaret, volunteer)

Next we come to the difficulty over how directive volunteers should be – how willing they should be to tell callers what to do.

Volunteer helplines make no pretence (and should make no pretence) about the nature and extent of the training given to volunteers. There is no body of knowledge handed down from an eminent forerunner upon which to base current volunteer practice, there is no worldwide governing council sitting in judgement on the standards of any individual volunteer. Rather there is the day-to-day collective wisdom of working volunteers passed to one another by both formal and informal methods, regulated pragmatically rather than by a professional code or authoritarian imposition.

Directive or non-directive?

One issue which seems to divide the professional counselling world is particularly important in the work of volunteer gay helplines. That is the issue of directive or non-directive counselling.

Put crudely, the distinction is between those who, as an article of faith and practice, *never* offer direction to a client, and those who see offering direction as *one* of the tools which a counsellor may choose to use as and when appropriate.

There would seem to be two different reasons for choosing to operate within a non-directive style of counselling. One of these rests on its value as a tool in counselling, the other relates to social acceptability. Because most gay helplines – and many other volunteer helplines too – claim to operate non-directively, it is worth considering the reasons for choosing to do so.

Margaret is working non-directively when she tries to create an environment in which Jane feels able to work through her own problems, and tries to work out a solution for herself. This is an environment in which Jane is empowered.

Advocates of non-directive methods argue that real and long-lasting benefits come only through the caller feeling able to make decisions, and feeling able to take responsibility for making those decisions, because only in these conditions will the caller be able to follow through to their conclusions the decisions she has made.

It is important in this situation that the caller understands that the volunteer and the helpline believe it to be wrong to give direction. If anyone else – the volunteer, for example – takes over any of these responsibilities, then the caller may continue to see herself as a victim, not as an individual, as a child, not as an adult.

It is easy, the argument goes, for a volunteer to offer advice. However, if sometime later, something goes 'wrong' in Jane's life in her own eyes, she may try to deny responsibility for her actions by blaming Margaret for the advice given and this may reinforce her view of herself as a victim. Alternatively, just as damaging, Jane may come to depend on Margaret because of her 'need' for advice.

Non-directive counselling can be applied in a less-than-pure form. There are those who operate with a non-dogmatic approach to non-directiveness. They reserve the right to offer advice where it seems appropriate and is not likely to create a dependency. They make clear the context in which any advice is being offered. They offer advice only when it would be unreasonable to persist with 'You must make your own decisions' in a 'cat-and-mouse' fashion.

Can a gay helpline be non-directive?

It can be argued that the mere existence of a *gay* helpline is directive. It directs the caller to the view that a gay alternative exists and that there are circumstances in which it is acceptable.

Some far-right Christians (so-called) have attempted, from time to time, to establish telephone 'counselling services' which deny that any gay alternative can ever be acceptable, but at no point could it be argued that these services operate non-directively.[8]

By contacting a *gay* helpline a caller can be presumed to expect that the helpline believes that there is an acceptable gay alternative. Some new volunteers are surprised to find that this is not always the case, there are still some callers who express amazement when a helpline is supportive of their gay feelings.

So, in the sense that a gay helpline has a perspective on the world – a view about the acceptability of gay lifestyles – it can be thought to be directive. This goes for any helpline which does not accept the status quo in society. Those who oppose its view can accuse it of being directive, and thereby pursue a claim that it is an unsuitable means of counselling anyone. This fails to understand the nature of directiveness and of counselling.

To give direction one must start from somewhere. But the parallel to that is that to be non-directive, counsellor and client must be sure of where each stands so that confidence can be built up between them. So to be non-directive, in a sense one must also start from somewhere.

In this context there is no reason why that starting point cannot be full acceptance of gay and lesbian equality. It is possible, therefore, for a helpline to be governed by a philosophy of its own and still be non-directive – still encourage self-determination – if it chooses *that* to be its counselling style. Non-directiveness is a style of counselling, not a statement of lack of purpose or direction. Indeed, support for gay and lesbian equality, a philosophy which emphasises self-determination, could be said to *require* a non-directive style of counselling.

Social acceptability

Apart from its value as a tool in counselling, the other major reason why many helplines insist that they use non-directive counselling concerns social approval.

Many helplines deal constantly with ideas, problems and issues which are only partially accepted in society at large. Indeed, if that were not the case there might be no need for them. Any organisation which deals with unaccepted or only partially accepted ideas, problems and issues must always be ready for attacks on it from those who find those matters offensive.

The recent attacks of Church and State upon support for gay and lesbian equality have already been considered. Physical attacks on premises occupied by gay helplines are not unknown;[9] verbal abuse from callers is so common that dealing with it forms a standard part of the training programme of most volunteers; and attacks on the value of the service offered by gay helplines in the form of hate mail, abusive calls and worse, occur from time to time. It is these attacks on the value of the service which are relevant here.

Many of the critics claim that gay helplines exist to 'pervert' people (especially the young) – or to 'intentionally promote homosexuality' – or (and this is seen in the same negative way by the critics), to 'recruit' people to 'homosexuality'.

The absence of any criticism of detailed working methods of gay helplines, even by social services personnel who might feel able to offer reasoned criticism, is remarkable and may reflect well on standards. However it may be that those who are in a position to constructively criticise refrain from doing so, in case they are thought to be supporters of the 'moral majority'.

It is not possible to convince those who have closed minds, but it does seem that to be able to claim that the style with which a helpline operates is a non-directive one convinces some of the less closed-minded.

There are two qualifications which must be made to that. First, it is not clear whether such a claim really does convince, or whether it merely allows social services officers to sound authoritative and professional in their defence of a helpline which has had the temerity to apply for funding from a local authority.

Second, detractors make test calls. Detractors have difficulty in finding evidence to condemn those helplines which maintain careful record systems and have a style which refuses to direct people in what they should do.

It is detrimental to a helpline – and to volunteers' views of the service they offer – that it should adopt a style of counselling merely to fend off ill-informed attacks. To operate with non-directive methods simply to deter attackers may be easy to understand but it demonstrates a lack of self-confidence. The argument runs like this: to be able to offer some assistance, even if it means using (or seeming to use) a counselling style in which we do not believe, but which is socially acceptable, is a small price to pay to avoid being prevented from offering any assistance at all.

At the level of the individual volunteer the matter is different. Non-directive styles have much merit, particularly through their refusal to allow the caller to act as a 'victim' all the time. However, some volunteers adopt non-directive styles because they do not have sufficient self-confidence; they are frightened of the consequences of offering 'wrong' advice. Where this is the case additional training often leads the volunteer away from the lack of self-confidence and allows him or her to recognise the worth of their own views, and therefore to feel able to offer advice.

It is only when the volunteer feels strong enough to offer advice that she/he will be able to make a reasoned judgement about whether to use non-directive styles, or will be able to participate in helpline discussions on the matter.

'Can I answer anybody or only people like me?'

The caller was a sergeant in the army and very proud of it. He has been married and has three sons, all of them 'real men', in the army. Now he wants to have sex with someone like himself. I am a pacifist, and against all male machismo, and I don't want to encourage his militaristic views. I have nothing in common with him, how can I help him? (Neville, volunteer)

From within a humanitarian perspective the existence of gay helplines – separate from general helplines like the Samaritans – requires the belief that assisting people with particular problems requires specialist knowledge of those problems, and of the environment in which those problems are experienced.

This argument applies whether the specialist knowledge concerns gay and lesbian matters or race or disability and has been used to justify the development of helplines within each of these fields separate from the general helplines. It has also been used to justify the setting up of helplines dealing with marriage and problems surrounding it, and helplines dealing with the effects of particular medical conditions.

There are those who would take the argument one stage further and insist that only those who have experienced for themselves social oppression can be of assistance to others similarly oppressed; only the oppressed may empower other oppressed people.

How far can these arguments be taken? In Britain, who helps wheelchair-bound 55-year-old married lesbians of Irish origin? Other lesbians? Other married lesbians? Other lesbians of Irish origin? Other wheelchair-bound lesbians? Gay men? Wheelchair-bound 55-year-old married gay men of Irish origin?

The direct sharing of experience is a very valuable tool in assisting the personal development of anyone if the recipient can see that the experience is relevant. If the relevance of the experience is unclear to the caller, it may not empower, rather it may cause increased isolation.

For example, it may be valuable in relieving his isolation to tell a coalminer that there are other gay men who are coalminers. It may also be valuable to say that a conversation with one could easily be arranged, but the meeting may be disastrous to the caller's self-esteem if he decides that what he has in common is of little consequence because the other miner is good-looking and he, the caller, is ugly.

Shared experience needs to be generalised experience, shared feelings and attitudes, rather than sharing details of personal life, because the sharing is only valuable if thereby fears and apprehensions are allowed to emerge so that personal growth may be achieved. Shared experience of personal details is of only limited benefit in achieving this objective, and it has attendant dangers.

Generalised life experience

- Can volunteers on gay helplines answer calls from people of the opposite sex?
- Can people who have not experienced (in one form or another) the social oppression of gay men and lesbian women answer calls to a gay helpline?
- Does a helpline need to have black or Asian volunteers before it can answer calls from black or Asian callers?
- Does a helpline need volunteers who have been married to deal with callers experiencing problems concerning their marriages?

As with many of these issues, there are several influences which helplines balance. One of these influences – common humanity – seeks to play down the need to share any specific experiences, even to the extent of recognising that over-identification of the caller with a particular volunteer may be harmful. If callers, in the process of developing self-assurance, see their volunteer as being the walking embodiment of the solutions to all problems, then the search for solutions to their own problems is likely to be arrested.

However, the view which emerges from a liberationist perspective is rather different. The test of a potential volunteer is not that they should be the same as the caller in any particular aspect, but that they have a good understanding of the nature of the oppressions under which people struggle – or that they are, as it were, 'in good standing in the liberationist faith'. Where 'the faith' contains matters concerning group identity then the similarity between volunteer and caller must be adhered to. So, for example, a black consciousness-raising helpline could not have white volunteers and a helpline committed to helping women from a feminist perspective could not have male volunteers.

Within the gay context this general principle is adhered to more or less strictly. In the stricter version, since the liberation concerns not only matters to do with same-sex relationships but also matters to do with the place of women in society, woman must answer woman, man must answer man, and all volunteers must have direct personal experience of the oppression of gay people. If people who do not personally identify as gay wish to be involved in the work of these helplines, they may assist in fund raising, running jumble sales or even making tea, but they must not be telephone volunteers.

Even in this strict version there is often a recognition of the part that parents of gay men and lesbian women, or spouses, may play in matters concerning other parents or other spouses.

The less strict version of adherence to this principle permits those who have personal experience of the oppression of gay men and lesbian women which is not direct, such as parents or spouses, to become volunteers. It needs to be clear, however, that such people have had to cope with some break in their lives because of social disapproval of gay or lesbian sexual identity – at home, at work or at play.

From the point of view of the gay scene, the primary objective of a helpline is to incorporate the caller as easily as possible into some part of the gay world. Incorporation is going to be easier if there is a certain matching of characteristics of volunteer and caller – so professional to professional, trade unionist to trade unionist, disco enthusiast to disco enthusiast. From this point of view, since those who do not see themselves as gay are not part of the gay world, they cannot be members of a helpline – though they may become involved in satellites of the gay world, in 'parents of gays' groups, for example.

The real world of the helpline

Many helplines are collectively less conscious of the reasons for the decisions they take than this analysis might suggest, for volunteers are essentially caring pragmatists. Taking the issue of non-gay telephone volunteers, for example, most of the small number who are involved work in small-town helplines, and almost all have specialist knowledge or direct personal experience of gay oppression.

Most larger helplines, those with, say, 30 or more volunteers, deliberately seek recruits from those who face discrimination for other reasons, such as race or disability. This permits all volunteers to learn more about these forms of discrimination and to keep up to date with ways in which they may be combated. It also means that the helpline is in a position to cross-refer callers who wish to be introduced to the gay world, so that the caller finds acquaintances and friends who share his or her interests and concerns.

Much training time with volunteer recruits is spent in helping them to see that exchange of direct experience is only one of many means of assistance which may be offered. Volunteers often need to see that it is not the details of their own experience which may be helpful to the caller, rather it is in identifying the feelings present in those experiences.

For example, it is not the experience of having a lover walk out that is important, it is the experience of having to work through rejection, loneliness, grief, whatever events have caused these emotions. In developing their awareness to others with different experiences, trainee volunteers learn how to listen rather than talk.

The common thread in helpline policy on this matter seems to be not so much 'I am not like you', but 'Whatever our apparent differences in experience and life, I am like you, so let us see how we can share to our mutual benefit'. There are examples of breakdown of this sentiment, and this issue will be considered when assessing the quality of the work of helplines in chapter 7.

5 Callers and their World

In chapter 3 we considered three basic questions which are asked frequently of helplines, questions which concerned the caller alone. Now we move on to issues which cause serious problems in callers' relationships with other people and the world around them. Four issues are considered here: 'Should I tell my parents that I am lesbian/gay?', 'Should I tell my spouse; what about my children?', 'Should I be faithful to my lover?' and 'Will I fit into the gay world?'

'Should I tell my parents?'

Dealing with questions concerning disclosures takes up a large proportion of volunteers' time. The questions concern a wide range of areas of life and are not limited to relations between parents and children. Other areas include disclosure between marriage partners (considered on pages 74–78), and between workmates. Here we shall concentrate on relationships between children and their parents, but first we will move away from gay-related issues and consider some other examples.

Some pictures of relationships

- 'I am pregnant,' says the unmarried teenage daughter to her parents.
- 'I have joined the Moonies', declares the sixth-former to his parents.

Either of these statements might cause any reaction from violence, rejection or stunned silence through to loving acceptance or dismissive lack of interest. The making of such a statement precedes, and causes, a change in the social relationships within the family.

An otherwise prudish father and mother now have to cope with knowing that their daughter has been having pre-marital sex; that she has failed to take adequate precautions against pregnancy; and that she has failed to have a quick abortion, which would (at least) have relieved her of the pain of admitting pregnancy to her parents and which would have relieved them of the need to cope with this situation.

They think they have failed. They feel that they have not educated their daughter properly, either on the matter of precautions, or on the place of sex within marriage. They feel rejected.

Church-going parents who brought up their children in the church are now aware that their son, whom they thought shared their religious views, has joined a controversial sect, and will be leaving home to join that sect in its strange lifestyle.

They think they have failed. Their whole lives have been centred round the church and on giving their children a good Christian upbringing. They are torn about what to do. On the one hand they feel that their son should be allowed the right to his own opinions and beliefs, but on the other hand they do not want him to be taken away by people whom they see as evil. They feel that they have failed to teach their son what is right, and have failed to take enough notice of him to anticipate this development. They feel rejected.

Three major reactions to failure emerge from looking at situations like these. Reject the evidence is the first: 'You're not really pregnant'; 'They have brainwashed him'.

Accept failure and reorganise life around a recognition of the failure is the second. Perhaps in these two cases this reaction would be: 'Things have gone wrong, but she is still our daughter and the baby will be our grandchild' and 'It is his decision, we must respect him for making it and pray for his future'.

The third reaction is to redefine success and failure so that the failure is no longer a failure: 'At long last we can admit that she was born out of wedlock too, and nowadays half of all first babies are conceived out of wedlock, so let's make sure she attends all the ante-natal classes' and 'We really must read about this new religion, perhaps it is more relevant today for young people than our church'.

Another example concerns a 22-year-old man who returns home having been to hospital for tests. Unknown to his parents, with whom he lives, he has been having difficulties with his limbs and the feeling in them. The diagnosis of multiple sclerosis comes after many hospital visits. How does he tell his parents? What does he tell them? Does he tell them anything?

Going through his mind are thoughts such as 'Perhaps, even after all these tests, the diagnosis is still wrong', 'Perhaps they will find a cure for it before things become too obvious', 'Perhaps they have already noticed', or 'Perhaps the doctor has already told them despite her promise not to'.

The immediate reaction of the parents, particularly if they have had no warning, may be one of failure, guilt, hopelessness or despair. Of these, failure and guilt seem to be the easiest to dispel when the nature of the medical condition is explained to them, and, in particular, when they realise that he has not 'caught it' either from them or through some negligence on their part.

These pictures allow us to place the gay disclosure issue into context. It must be recognised that the gay issue has similarities with other disclosure issues, and that consideration of disclosure requires an examination of relationship between parents and children.

Helpline volunteers produce many varied examples of disclosure stories, each with its own nuances. However, let two stories suffice: Christine and her parents, and Eric and his aged mother.

Christine and her parents

Imagine a family consisting of four – father, mother, girl of nineteen (Christine) and boy of seventeen. The parents believe in 'live and let live'. The 19-year-old girl contacts a helpline with the question 'Should I tell my parents?' What are the influences surrounding any advice a volunteer would offer?

What to tell, and why

It is simple to respond to the question 'Should I tell my parents?' with a reflex gay liberation response, 'Yes, come out', echoing the Gay Liberation Front slogan of the early 1970s. For many volunteers it is even easier to talk callers out of any such action. Volunteers, in the main, have many friends 'on the gay scene' and many voices there deride 'coming out' as having no benefits and as destroying the semi-secret enjoyment of a partially separate gay or lesbian world. However, their training helps the volunteers to take this question seriously, to stand aside from gay liberation slogans and derisive gay bar talk.

Volunteers, then, are seeking to balance these factors with their training and instincts to act in a humanitarian way. This involves helping callers to weigh up their own needs and the needs of their families, and empowering them to take their own decisions.

The volunteer needs to assess the level of risk to relationships which each caller is prepared to take, and needs to develop strategies to assist callers with those risks. That involves helping callers to consider the depth and strength of the relationships within their families.

In the example given above, has Christine ever kept any other major matter concerning her life secret from them, or, conversely, does the family ever discuss anything intimate?

With considerations of depth and strength go feelings of trust. How deeply does Christine care what her parents think? Is her apparent concern to tell them merely skin deep? Underneath, is she prepared to be thrown out of her home, even willing to use their reaction to being told as an excuse for leaving the family?

So the volunteer and Christine may work towards some common understanding of why she wants to tell her parents that she is lesbian. But they also have to consider what it is that the caller means to tell her parents.

Does Christine want to tell her parents that she is confused about sexuality? Is the proposed statement 'I am a lesbian' really a code for 'I cannot cope with boys, therefore I must be a lezzie', or even 'All my friends have boyfriends. I am always left out, therefore I must be lesbian'.

Alternatively, perhaps Christine wants to tell her parents about her exploration of sex and sexuality and the conclusion she has drawn. Without careful planning, however, it is most unlikely that her parents will understand her statement 'I am a lesbian' to mean:

I have spent a great deal of time working through my feelings and attitudes towards other people, to sexuality, to gender and to sex. I have come to the conclusion that for me at this time the most appropriate and most enjoyable lifestyle is in the company of other women who, like myself, enjoy emotional and sexual relationships with people of our own sex.

though that might well be what she wants to say.

A third – and apparently simpler – alternative is that Christine wants to introduce her girlfriend to her parents in the general hope and expectation that their reaction would be similar to the one they would have if it were a boyfriend Christine was introducing to them.

What response?

How will Christine's parents interpret her words: 'I am a lesbian'? Alongside thinking about what she means, Christine and the volunteer working with her may need to consider what meanings each of her parents will give to the words. What overtones have words like 'lesbian', 'gay', 'homosexual' got for them? Are there overtones in their minds of promiscuous whores, pneumatic-drill-wielding dragons, ferocious women corrupting young girls, or have they developed more positive views?

'Lesbian', 'gay' and 'homosexual' are words which have attracted a variety of responses. Some people have very strange ideas of what these words mean, and this is not assisted by their confusion which surrounds the 'be/do' debate. Christine may need to be aware of these responses, these ideas and these confusions, in order that she does not unwittingly find herself dealing with issues entirely unconnected with what she wants to tell her parents.

The volunteer working with Christine balances all the influences on her and tries to steer a course which empowers Christine to see what it is she wants to disclose and why. Thereby she helps Christine assess the possible reactions and weigh up the risks and benefits to her relations with her family, so that she may pursue a course of action which will assist her and will not cause unnecessary harm to others.

Eric and his aged mother

'My mother must never find out that I have been talking to you. She is 80 years old and it would kill her.' So speaks a 45-year-old man who lives at home with his widowed mother, has never married, and has spent a great deal of time looking after his mother in the last few years.

Eric met Fred many years ago. Fred is in his late thirties. They first met in a public lavatory where both of them were seeking a casual sexual encounter. The casual encounter was repeated many times and they gradually became friends. Now the friendship between them is faltering because Eric continues to insist on deceiving his mother.

But there is another view. It might indeed kill her, but she might die happy if she felt that, after all these years, her son had finally decided to trust her with his big secret. She may have known for many years that he had a big secret, and feared far worse than this 'sex with men'. Perhaps, if only she had the chance to meet Fred, she might be pleased that Eric was happy with this special friend he has found.

Sometimes the volunteer needs to help the caller consider whether the insult to a parent in *not* discussing things with them is not much harder for her to bear than the difficulties associated with coping with the gay issue.

The volunteer

Disclosure calls put a tremendous strain on some volunteers, and in particular on those who have not 'come out' to their own family and friends.

Many helplines impose the rule on aspiring volunteers that they must have dealt with all their own disclosure problems before being trained as volunteers, but some helplines (mostly those outside large centres of population) feel they cannot impose such rules.

For those volunteers who have not made their own disclosures there are problems of relating to the caller's desire to look seriously at that possibility. A volunteer's own problems in that area may make it very difficult to listen attentively to the caller. Conversely, a volunteer who appears very confident about 'being out' runs the risk, albeit unwittingly, of being seen as a threat by callers. Volunteers need to be responsive to callers' needs and should not, unnecessarily, increase their disquiet.

'What about my marriage and children?'

Moving from disclosures by children to their parents, let us consider two marriages, that between Mike and Rosalind, and that between Julia and Robert.

Mike and Rosalind

Mike and Rosalind are in their mid-thirties and have been married 10 years, with two kids aged 8 and 6. Mike is having an affair with another man. Rosalind is getting increasingly suspicious of his 'business trips', and suspects he is having an affair with another woman. He has denied that, but the marriage relationship is suffering.

When Mike telephones the gay helpline to talk about the conflict he is feeling about his marriage to Rosalind and his relationship with David, and about the rows he is expecting, he is making an important statement merely by making the telephone call. Most people with marriage difficulties who think of contacting an agency or helpline will be aware of the services of the marriage advisory groups, such as Relate (formerly the Marriage Guidance Council) for example.

In telephoning a gay helpline rather than a marriage advisory service Mike is likely to be placing the 'gay' part of the issue above the 'marriage' part, and this may herald an intention to take what he may see as the 'gay' route out of the difficulty (leaving Rosalind for David).

Mike's question 'Should I tell my wife?' raises the same issues as before: Why tell? What to tell? How will she respond?, but with one additional concern: What about the kids?

The matter of marriage breakdown presents far more consequential effects than does disclosure to parents. To deal with Mike carefully, the volunteer has to explore with him all the dimensions of the marriage relationship and alternatives to it. That may mean that the call is best followed through by someone who has contact with both partners. Many callers find it too difficult to work through these matters, and volunteers often find either that callers have (precipitately) separated from the wives or have submerged their feelings for the 'other man', ditching him without explanation.[1]

Early gay liberation and some strands of feminism have expounded on the outdated nature of heterosexual pairing and its inherent oppression and have urged all to leave their marriage partners. On the other hand bar talk (a good indicator of the temperature of the male gay world) points to the number of marriages 'saved' because the man is able to go off from time to time for 'sexual relief' with another man, or men.

The volunteer who is seeking to empower Mike will be ensuring that his empowerment includes his recognition that he cannot exploit Rosalind and David. Therefore the volunteer will help him to consider the option of leaving Rosalind for David alongside two other options. One of these is the option of working through the issues with Rosalind and coming to a new understanding of the nature of their marriage. The other is the option of supressing his feelings for David and ending the relationship.

Julia and Robert

Volunteers have to deal with all sorts of horror stories, such as eviction when the landlord finds you are gay, summary dismissal from employment without any recourse in law because your employer does not want to employ lesbians, parents declaring that they never want to see their child again.

Each of these stories represents a dimension of the unthinking hostility which still exists in society – an unthinking hostility backed by fear, an unthinking hostility backed by government.[2] However half-hearted government support for existing race equality and sex equality legislation may seem to many, and however inadequate the Acts have been in eliminating discrimination, those Acts are on the statute books.

Not only is there no such similar Act concerning gay men and lesbians, there are many instances of courts and tribunals upholding as reasonable outrageous discrimination against lesbians and gay men in the fields such as housing and employment.[3]

The effects these horror stories have on those who hear them vary. Some simply claim not to believe the stories, and carry on as before without taking any account of the institutionalised discrimination and public hostility which such stories indicate. Some are made more resentful of a hostile society and retreat further into a ghetto, hoping thereby to avoid the consequences for them. Some are made angry and become involved in campaigns of one sort or another designed to combat the discrimination or hostility.

Others take the stories to heart and are affected profoundly, their self-esteem is reduced (still further), and they retreat into themselves, unable to handle the matters presented to them. Both men and women are affected in all these ways, but some horror stories have widespread consequences for the self-esteem of some women. The stories affect their self-esteem as women, and affect their self-esteem as lesbians.

The worst horror stories, many volunteers report, are those concerning women having their children forceably removed from them by an irate ex-husband backed by a court order from a judge who has declared that he regards lesbians as disgusting perverts.[4]

It is not clear just how many cases like this there have been. In one sense it does not matter. What matters is that there is a widely held perception (held both by lesbians at large and by helpline volunteers) that such instances are widespread.[5]

The fear is one which has great strength. The fear that a hostile and deeply prejudiced legal system will enforce itself on a woman to the extent of forceably removing her children from her brings together many of the concerns felt by women callers when calling a helpline.

These are concerns about the conflicts between motherhood and lesbianism, about the heavy hand of the law violating one's own private space, about rejecting marriage and about being rejected by society. They are concerns shared by other women who are seeking to empower themselves, to stand up against men when society seems to require otherwise.

Julia and Robert had been married for seven years. She was 30, he 37. She had not been married before, he had one marriage under his belt and had fathered two children now in the custody of their mother. There was one child of this marriage, Timothy, aged five.

Julia had only slowly become aware of her wish for an emotional and sexual relationship with another woman. For some time she had been loosely connected with a women's group and she had read a lot about women's rights. Robert did not (superficially at least) expect her to stay in the home to look after children. Indeed as soon as Timothy was old enough to go to nursery school, Julia returned to work with Robert's encouragement.

She knew he was having affairs with other women. It was not spoken about and she did not find the idea too awful at first. She felt that this gave her the freedom to develop friendships in her women's health group.

Her friendship with Helen had been growing for almost a year before they admitted to one another that each had become attached emotionally to the other. As their relationship developed Julia ensured that Timothy got to know and like his new Auntie Helen.

Then came the awful moment. Robert came home drunk one evening and accused her of having an affair with Helen. She did not deny it. He had a number of gay friends and was never abusive about their sexuality. She accused him of having a series of mistresses. He too, did not deny it. He walked out and went to stay with his latest mistress.

The next thing she knew was when Robert started custody proceedings over Timothy. He had lost two children in a previous custody case, and was determined not to lose another this time. He was prepared to use every trick in the book to get custody of Timothy.

Julia's legal advisers told her that Robert would get custody if the lesbian issue was brought before the judge.[6] They were clear also that the judge might even refuse her access to her son. Her only hope was an out-of-court arrangement which gave Robert custody but which agreed access arrangements. She could not win.

Her husband, who walked straight into the arms of his mistress, was a right and proper father who could be given custody. She was a disgusting pervert who was not fit to mother a child. Robert would get Timothy despite general agreement that, other things being equal, a child should go to its mother.

The helpline was faced with two women at their wits' end. Julia was beginning to doubt her own capabilities as a mother, and her self-esteem as a woman had taken a serious battering.

If only she had realised it, Julia was being faced with the choice of motherhood versus lesbian identity. She could not see why, in a rational society, she should have to make that choice. Nor could the volunteer.

Helen felt guilty because she felt she had been the cause of Julia losing Timothy. She wanted Julia to offer to return to Robert. She even offered to agree never to see Julia again.

The volunteer had the distressing task of helping the callers pick up the pieces after an injustice had been done to them which she could not explain or justify. It was an injustice which attacked the very roots of lesbian strength and women's rights. The volunteer has to cope with her own anger and frustration, and still be able to help the caller to work through her feelings.

None the less the support which the helpline could provide could not immediately right the wrong all agreed had been perpetrated on Julia and Timothy. The helpline provided Julia and Helen with friendship and with understanding, and with details of campaigning and self-help groups organised around the lesbian custody issue.

The helpline's women's support group was able to provide both women with an opportunity to talk over in an empathetic environment the hurt each felt, and the guilt which Helen (in particular) felt. They also helped Julia prepare for, and enjoy, the access she had to Timothy and helped her cope after each occasion had ended.

'Should I be faithful to my lover?'

Many people feel themselves to be subject to two apparently conflicting pressures within their personal lives: to 'have a good time' and be seen to have a good time, and to seek an ideal relationship and to settle for nothing else. Helplines often find callers want to talk through their own personal conflicts and it is these conflicts to which I now turn.

The models which we have to look up to are very important for our day-to-day living. These may be parent, teacher, work supervisor, film star or television personality. Most likely we will have a large number of people on whom we model ourselves, and we take bits from each of them to help us build up our lifestyle.

'Being gay' has been hidden for a very long time, and as with other oppressed groups, being hidden means losing one's history. Liberation includes the development of group history – black history, women's history, gay men's history.[7]

The separate gay social world to be found in most large centres has only been apparent for less than 20 years. Therefore many young people who see themselves as gay feel that they have few appropriate gay role models to emulate. Of course it may be that this very lack of social conventions (and lack of role models) attracts some people, but at some point models emerge and are held in high regard within any new community.

The most obvious model might seem to be boy and girl meet and fall in love, they get married and have children and live happily together for the rest of their lives. But what use is that model to the young gay adult? If, for example, a young man is expecting to live a life of relating sexually – for the most part – with other men, what style of life should he seek? Should he seek a gay equivalent of 'boy meets girl', the 'boy meets boy' model?

The dream – boy meets boy, John and Richard

John and Richard have been having an emotional and sexual relationship for over a year, or (to put it another way) John has been going out with his boyfriend, Richard, for over a year. While still wanting to have a relationship with Richard, John also wants to have casual sex with people he meets in gay pubs and clubs from time to time. While this playing around does not seem to bother his friend, John is sufficiently uneasy about it that he telephones the helpline to ask for advice.

The wide range of relationship styles within the male gay scene is clear to most young gay men very soon after they become involved. It ranges from frequent episodes of casual recreational sex with many partners (usually unknown to one another) through to intentionally monogamous couples.[8]

John's straight (heterosexual) friends will be acquainted with this range of styles too, though the proportions involved in each style may be rather different. A life of frequent casual encounters is far from unknown in straight circles, particularly for those under 30, but for older people it is far less common than in the gay male world.

There is one lifestyle which seems far more common in the gay male world than in straight circles. That is to have a series (one after the other) of one- or two-year relationships, in each of which there is space for occasional sex outside the relationship.

In calling the helpline, John is expressing his unease about his relationship and where it fits into the range. He may also be expressing unease about his friendship with Richard. Perhaps he has seen Richard as the 'boy of his dreams', and his desire for casual sex with other people may mark a change in the way he sees Richard.

The dream and its consequences

It would seem that the dream of a lover for life is very widespread in gay male circles. However, John and Richard may separate in circumstances where a married couple with children would be likely to spend time trying to work through their difficulties rather than end their relationship. There are rarely legal and financial ties in the typical gay male relationship, and few partners have direct responsibility for children.

A separation allows John and Richard to have second attempts at finding their dream, and a third, and a fourth attempt, and so it seems to go on. Each separation may be accompanied by traumatic events in the lives of those concerned, and may be met by cynical responses from friends. These responses may serve to reduce still further the impetus to sort out difficulties which many married couples might regard as commonplace and soluble in the compromise of personalities which forms a marriage.

The impact of AIDS and HIV infection is affecting the attitudes of many gay men towards relationships.[9] It seems to be that, at least for the duration of AIDS as a major uncontained health risk and at least in those regions where it has become a day-by-day issue for gay men, fear of the consequences of becoming HIV antibody positive is acting as some sort of counterbalance, and is producing a greater willingness to sort out differences within relationships.

So John and Richard face two pressures: to have a good time (within the constraints of possible HIV infection), and to seek an ideal relationship. Underlying these pressures is a failure of the gay male world to reach a consensus on the purpose of sexual relationships.

Sexual acts conventionally have been seen to have three purposes, and the ideal state is said to be when all three are found in one relationship:

- that sex is the mechanism by which the species creates its own succession

- that sex is one means by which relationships are sustained
- that sex is for pleasure

Any relationship between two people of the same sex is biologically prevented from resulting in children (though some gay couples do parent and nurture children, often where one of the couple is the biological parent of the children). This leaves the remaining two purposes. John is struggling to find his own acceptable compromise between them: between sex for pleasure and sex as a means by which relationships are nurtured.

The volunteer and John

In his struggle to find his own compromise, John has telephoned the helpline. The volunteer tries to help John work through his feelings while taking account of the pressures which exist, both on John and on the volunteer.

Liberation ideals push in two different directions. One direction emphasises how new is positive gay identity, declaring that therefore there are great opportunities for the re-examination of all relationship roles, and indeed other matters such as gender roles and the ways in which parts of society fit together.

The other direction presents a positive gay identity as something which has a history and which can claim important figures in the past who can be seen as models for our lives today.

The best known institutions to present this view have been the gay theatre company, Gay Sweatshop[10] (which since the mid-1970s has presented plays about the gay community often linking contemporary struggles for acceptance with past struggles) and the Hall-Carpenter Historical Archive.[11] This archive commemorates in its title, the famous lesbian writer, Radclyffe Hall, and the gay socialist thinker, Rev Edward Carpenter. The archive, in its efforts to unearth and preserve material relating to lesbian and gay matters over many years, has helped develop a sense of community history.

These strands must be assessed alongside the hedonism (selfish pleasure-seeking) of much of the gay (male) world and John must be assisted towards developing his own personal position. He must be empowered to stand apart from over-bearing hedonism in order to develop his own approach in which he neither exploits nor is exploited.

There are many examples of exploitation. These include gay men who make high-minded statements about relationships, but practise something different. Richard appears to be John's primary concern, and if his relationship with Richard does not figure in his resolution of the matter, then both John and Richard will be demeaned in the process.

The volunteer and his/her own life

John's question 'Should I be faithful to my lover?' is poignant because he is, in a way, seeking permission to abandon a gay equivalent of 'boy meets girl', permission to adopt the most common gay male lifestyle: a relationship with one other man with an acceptance on both parts that sexual encounters of a casual recreational nature with others, known or unknown, may take place. Male helpline volunteers may well be party to this lifestyle themselves.

Therefore, calls relating to difficulties with relationships may place the volunteer under some emotional strain. Like other issues considered in this book, this question may bring a male volunteer face-to-face with difficulties which are recurrent in many gay men's lives, and his training as a volunteer will be called into question if he is unable to distance himself from John and allow him to consider his own position. The male caller may well believe that there will be another Prince Charming round the corner. In order to avoid colluding with the caller, the male volunteer will need to resist the pressures on him from all directions.

'Will I fit into the gay world?'

Moving to a new job, moving to a new area, joining a new club – each of these experiences brings with it a degree of apprehension. Two examples may be helpful.

Linda, aged 19, lived and worked in a small town over 20 miles from the nearest meeting place for lesbians. She had telephoned the helpline and spoken to a volunteer on three occasions, agreeing on the third occasion to the suggestion from the volunteer that they meet at a coffee bar in Linda's town. The volunteer, Susan, found that the major problem on Linda's mind was 'Will I fit in? I don't live there. I have to travel. Perhaps the other lesbians will think that I am stupid, or ugly, or not worth talking to.'

Martin, aged 28 and rather shy, knew where the gay clubs and pubs were before he telephoned the helpline. He even seemed happy about being gay, but afraid of rejection. He asks Tim, the volunteer, 'What will I say? What do I do if they are all screaming queens? What do I do if someone tries it on with me? I am too old to be a teenager, so if I let on that I don't know what goes on, then will I be taken for a ride?'

These fears are very real. Helplines must not dismiss them.

Conformity

Most of us want to be like those around us: we want to conform socially. A few, however, consciously shun conformity. Most of us are not conscious of conforming socially, but when we cease to conform, for whatever reason, we are often made very aware of it. If we are seeking social conformity and it eludes us, it becomes a problem and we may find ourselves working harder and harder to achieve it.

While becoming aware that a gay sexuality is most suited to them, young people often feel isolated from other young people. Some withdraw into a private world. Some attack the world in which they live. Some attacks are very destructive – on persons or property – but most are characterised by rudeness, rejection of those people who accept them or rejection of the symbols of the society – schools, examinations and jobs. The rejection and isolation may instead lead to the young person finding for themselves a new social world, usually within some part of a recognisable gay world.

(Finding an acceptable new world after rejection – however caused – is not peculiar to young gay people. It is also found among those who feel rejected through, for example, being disabled, or on grounds of race or sex. In these cases, too, the new world will consist in the main of those who also feel rejected – others who are disabled, or of the same sex, or the same racial group.)

Helplines and social rejection

How do helplines try to assist those who feel socially isolated and rejected because of 'being gay'? For the most part helplines try to teach callers how to thrive – or at least exist – in a gay social environment.

(Lesbians and gay men who are 'out' to heterosexual friends are often asked by them why it is that they socialise in gay social facilities. For some the answer is about the search for new sexual contacts, or the search for a long-term partner, but for most the answer is about avoiding hostility in a natural environment. For two lovers to sit with arms round each other in a 'straight' pub would invite physical violence, summary expulsion, or (at best) abuse – even though between two lovers of opposite sex, this behaviour would cause no adverse comment. If one openly discussed matters concerning friends and the gay community it is likely that eavesdropping patrons would make complaints to licensees.)

As a first step the volunteers often try to fit the caller into their existing local gay-related social facilities, such as pubs, clubs and organisations.

So Tim and Susan help Linda and Martin to learn to enjoy the social facilities of the area.[12] Linda has to travel a long distance and so must plan her visits accordingly, and Martin has to pluck up a great deal of courage to meet anyone.

The speed at which Linda and Martin are introduced to these new places, and to new people, is a matter which Tim and Susan (with Martin and Linda) judge carefully, and most callers like Linda and Martin find their own level. However, there are some callers who find existing social environments uncomfortable and, for them, there may be a case for creating alternative facilities or pressurising existing social facilities to change.

Some helplines, particularly those who do not see themselves as counselling services, are content to give callers the names and addresses of pubs, clubs and organisations on request and leave to chance whether the caller fits into any of them. Others, particularly those of the FRIEND tradition, feel more of a sense of direct responsibility for their callers and so the volunteer will usually offer to take the caller to social venues and introduce him or her to them.

Gay-related social facilities – the typical region

Before looking at the merits of the approaches taken by various helplines to the existing gay social facilities, it may be useful to describe the nature and extent of the social facilities in a typical region, say the mythical region whose helplines were described in chapter 1.

In the regional centre there are four 'gay pubs'. These are public houses where the vast majority of the clientele are gay men or lesbian women and where casual visitors will fairly soon become aware of that. Of the four pubs, one is used almost exclusively by women. In the other three, if there are women present, the majority of them will be groups of women, and few will be mixing with men, though there is likely to be a great deal of casual friendliness expressed between groups of men and groups of women. Where couples are having private or intimate conversations most of the couples will be of the same sex.

Unlike working-men's clubs, which may also be exclusively male, an exclusively male gay pub will contain men of a variety of social backgrounds and ages, and, unlike many working-men's clubs, a large majority of those present will be under fifty.

One of the three men's pubs is different from the others in that it specialises in attracting those men who make a point of dressing in leather or in denim or in check shirts and jeans, or whatever is the current 'gay fashion' of the time. The other two pubs have a more general male clientele.

There are two gay clubs which open not long before pub closing times and will remain open into the early hours of the morning. A disco is an essential for both clubs, as is at least one bar. One of the clubs also provides a quieter area for those who wish to use the club as a late night social meeting place without the necessity of dancing or shouting over the disco music, or only exchanging glances because words are impossible or inappropriate. There is also a 'straight' night club which has hit hard times and has turned over one of its less popular nights to be a 'gay night'.

In addition to gay pubs and clubs, there are likely to be in each regional centre several non-commercial social groups. Some will owe their origins to a gay rights campaigning group, like the Campaign for Homosexual Equality or the Gay Liberation Front, or more recently, Stop the Clause Campaign Groups (named after the Wilshire/Knight amendment to the Local Government Act 1988): some will have origins in a college lesbian and gay students' society; some women-only groups may be based in a women's centre; and some will owe their origins to a gay helpline, established as a support group, perhaps for those who have difficulties socialising.

Political activity in any of these non-commercial groups had become – by the mid-1980s – almost non-existent except where a particular local issue arose. However, the impact of AIDS has created a new range of campaigning and social groups, and the efforts of David Wilshire and Dame Jill Knight to prevent local authorities from 'intentionally promoting homosexuality' has caused the biggest upsurge of political campaigning – and associated non-commercial socialising – since its heyday in the mid-1970s.

Social activity varies immensely from group to group. A few groups operate a wide-ranging social programme of theatre visits, visits to the swimming pool, coach trips to distant gay clubs and talks from visiting worthies. Even tupperware parties, whist drives and gay desert island discs have featured in the social programme of at least one group with a commendable history of political activism and social concern.[13]

Most non-commercial groups seem to consist of only a small core of people, many of whom have difficulties in large groups or pubs or clubs. The enthusiasm and commitment of the few keep the groups going, often without considering the value of the exercise.

Outside the regional centre, each of the four smaller centres of population has one pub which is widely used as a focus of the gay male (and, perhaps, lesbian) world. Unlike the pubs in the regional centre, some of these pubs are often 'mixed' (gay and straight). In these towns there is insufficient gay or lesbian-related business for a licensee to be prepared to reduce non-gay trade. Therefore there are unlikely to be any gay-related posters or notices.

In two of these four smaller centres there is also a non-commercial group. One of these has a large membership probably because of the discos it organises. There is also a small group of people who meet in a market town in a particularly rural part of the region. In such areas joining such a group is itself a political statement for many and, not unlike the early trade unions, provides some limited form of personal support for those who feel threatened by an apparently hostile world.

Helpline social groups

A sizeable minority of helplines have set up social groups, or acted as midwives for groups. Some of these groups have been for transvestites, some for the marriage partners of gay men or lesbian women, some for parents of gay or lesbian young people, some for those callers (many of them over 40) who have particular difficulty in mixing in.[14]

Setting up these support groups as alternative social groups is an article of faith for some helplines, fulfilling their aim to assist callers with any problem relating to the gay issue. For these helplines it does not matter too much if a support group dies as long as, during its lifetime, it has fulfilled a useful function for some people. Nor does it matter to the helpline – indeed it is often encouraged – if the support group separates itself from the helpline.

For some callers support groups become a permanent feature of their lives, for most they are a stepping stone into wider gay social circles. For a few at least they provide an opportunity to decide that the gay world has nothing to offer.

The last eight to ten years have seen the growth of a large

number of groups for young people emerging into adulthood – gay teenagers' groups. The majority of these are young gay men's groups, but they also include some young lesbian groups and some which claim (with greater or lesser veracity) to be genuinely mixed sex. Many of these owe their origins to helplines.

In almost every region there is a group of young people – perhaps with an age limit of 21, sometimes higher – who hold regular meetings where they can 'be themselves'; where sexual orientation is a membership card, not a bar.

Much has been written[15] about the problems of young gay men and young lesbian women, and there have been contributions from those concerned with gay teenagers' groups including members themselves, but there seems to be nothing from the perspective of the caring agency – the gay helpline.

A gay teenagers' group

It seems worthwhile to examine the founding and development of one gay teenage group. It is presented to show the ways in which such a development has contributed to, and been part of the work of a gay helpline. More than a dozen similar examples could have been chosen, each with its individual history and individual contribution to helpline work.

In the late 1970s, despair, annoyance and a feeling of failure filled one helpline's volunteers on realising – following an expansion of their telephone service – that more than fifty new callers appeared every month. Despair because over one quarter of the new callers were under 21; annoyance and frustration from some because these callers were felt to be difficult to handle and required a great deal of time and effort on the part of the volunteer; and a feeling of failure because the helpline seemed unable adequately to help this group of callers.

Driven by the enthusiasm of a few to devise new ways of helping the teenagers, and with the approval of all the volunteers, a group of the helpline's volunteers decided to plan a gay teenagers' group. The watchword was 'respectability', not because it was thought to be a desirable trait of a gay teenagers' group, nor because contact with 'the respectable' was thought likely to assist the young callers. Outsiders – professionals in social work, teaching, youth work, pastoral work – were included to give the venture 'credibility' in the face of a hostile world.

Of course only those outsiders thought to be enthusiastic supporters of the idea of a gay teenagers' group were included.

For some of them (gay and lesbian professional people), it was a way of identifying publicly with the gay world and a way of using their professional expertise to help young gay men and lesbian women sometimes without explicitly having to 'come out'.

Outsiders and helpline volunteers formed a management committee. Three people, two gay men and one lesbian woman, two of them helpline volunteers and the third a professional youth worker, were recruited to run the group, and general agreement was reached among the volunteers that where it was felt that a young person would benefit from meeting other young people in a 'safe' environment, callers under 21 should be referred to the new group.

Once a week in a town centre church hall, 5, 10, 20, later 30 or 40 teenagers, almost all male, met and did the things other teenagers do when they gather together. They played records, snooker and darts, they made and drank coffee, had discussions and arguments about all the things that teenagers talk about, including sex.

They talked about being gay, but not very often because it did not seem to matter once they were in the church hall. Everyone was gay, even the youth leaders. The youth leaders did the things youth leaders do when leading a group. They tried to involve the teenagers in making a video, in playing 'growth' games, in meaningful discussions about relationships, venereal disease (and later AIDS), or problems with parents.

Members of the management committee observed occasionally and asked questions. Some members of the group attended the bi-monthly management committee meetings (indeed the committee actively encouraged participation), and every year or two some of the teenagers would make a bid for power at these meetings.[16]

After about four years, through the enthusiasm generated by this group, another teenager group was established in one of the sub-regional centres, and later still another. A separate group for young lesbians was created within the overall ambit of a separate lesbian line and a women's centre.

The teenagers' group also had an associated parents' group which met from time to time. Its object was to allow parents to discuss their feelings on finding out that their son was gay or their daughter was lesbian. Some parents served on the management committee of the teenagers' group.

The group obtained some grant aid from the local education authority, and an associated housing project for housing teenagers evicted by their parents also obtained some council subsidy.

A teenagers' group and the helpline

Is it the responsibility of the helpline to protect the young from any excesses of the gay world? In setting up a teenagers' group is the helpline criticising the local gay social facilities?

The answer to both questions would seem to be 'yes', but the extent of the excess should not be overstated, nor should the level of criticism of the facilities. Indeed, the local facilities may benefit from such a group because since it exists commercial entrepreneurs have some means available to rid themselves of problem teenagers in their pubs and clubs.

Should gay teenagers be introduced to gay liberation ideas? From one point of view such groups could provide excellent opportunities for 'missionary' work on behalf of gay liberation. The helpline concerned in the example given has been keen to ensure that gay teenagers have some understanding of the recent history of gay rights in the UK, including the part played by more radical elements such as the Gay Liberation Front. Through most of its history the members of the teenagers' group (while agreeing) have set themselves against adopting any one perspective, but have from time to time become involved in campaigning about issues concerning lesbian and gay rights which have arisen in the area.

Will they fit in?

Linda and Martin will probably have to adjust their lifestyle to make them fit into the gay scene, at least to some extent.

One of them may not bother trying – perhaps deciding that he or she is not gay after all, or too ugly or too old – and so, withdraw from the gay world, or take up a place on its fringe. Only a minority of those people whom helplines introduce to gay-related social facilities are still part of that social environment after a year, but helplines have, so far, accepted that the major reasons for this concern the individual's ability to fit in. There seems little concern to examine the part which helpline volunteers play in this apparent failure.

Should the helpline expect them 'to fit in'? People's reasons for believing themselves to be gay are many and diverse. Commitment to the belief varies immensely. The gay world provides an environment in which people may test out their commitment to their belief and explore their reasons for that belief.

Acting within a caring framework, a helpline's responsibility is to try to prevent casualties, and one means of doing that is to extend the boundaries of the gay and lesbian worlds. The helpline may also see its role as providing the means by which callers may be integrated slowly into the existing social environment.

6 The More Difficult Problems

In addition to the issues of personal identity, relationships and socialising there are other issues which gay helpline volunteers face and which cause difficulties, such as psychiatric referrals – leading into referrals in general and relations with agencies of social control and social welfare; 'transvestism', with its apparent analogies with 'homosexuality'; and finally the issue of the sexual activities of callers. While not an exhaustive list of more serious problem issues facing gay helplines, these are considered here because each points to important components in the range of ideas, working practices and values which make up a helpline.

'We have an odd one here – what do I do?'

This man, he calls himself Norman, may be on the telephone every duty period – maybe more than once – taking up a line which other people may want to use, going over and over the same old set of 'problems' about how awful it is to be 'queer' as he calls it, and how everyone hates him because they can somehow tell he is a 'queer'. On and on he goes. Every volunteer on the helpline has tried to help him. What can we do? He is more than a nuisance, he is a nutter. (James, volunteer)

When and how do helplines extricate themselves from difficult calls? What do helplines do when a call becomes too difficult? Do they refer the caller to professionals, or are there alternative courses of action available?

Managing the odd one

The 'real weirdo nutter' is widely thought to be easy to

distinguish, and part of the self-proclaimed role of a helpline is to help all the rest. But where is the dividing line, indeed is there a dividing line? When does a problem become too difficult, and who helps then?

Every helpline has its callers like Norman, and worse. Even the most altruistic and long-suffering volunteer sometimes views such callers disparagingly. Often several helplines – both gay and general – in the same city have the same problem cases.

Helplines have different ways of handling these situations. One way is just to allow Norman to continue telephoning and hope that he will eventually give up or make some sense of what has been said to him. Helplines which have set their face against any sort of collective decision making often choose this course of action, by default. But in helplines where concern for the difficulties volunteers experience is as important as concern for the caller, some agreement on a strategy with such callers is often reached.

One such strategy, which seems to work, is for all such cases to be raised at the regular meeting of volunteers. Any volunteer may raise any case to demonstrate – usually by reference to notes made of the calls – that the caller is persistent and appears to be making little progress in making some sense of his or her own problems. It is then agreed that the caller is 'handed over' to one particular volunteer, Arthur for Norman, who agrees (alone) to deal with Norman's calls.

So, instead of Norman speaking to whichever volunteer happens to answer the telephone, when a volunteer realises that it is Norman on the telephone he or she tells him that Arthur is his 'personal' helpline volunteer, and when Arthur is next scheduled for duty. He or she then puts the telephone down, even though putting the telephone down on a caller is abhorred by many volunteers.

This strategy has several merits. It reduces the amount of time spent by volunteers on this caller, it reduces annoyance and frustration among volunteers caused by feeling that they are dealing at length with hopeless case after hopeless case, and it passes the caller on to one person.

Perhaps because the caller is no longer able to play one volunteer off against another, and can no longer go over and over the same problems with different volunteers, it is often the case that the nominated individual may be able to make some sort of progress.

Either Norman will decide that calling again is pointless (which is progress of a sort, if only for the helpline in ridding itself of him), or he will decide that things have begun to change and that problems are beginning to resolve themselves. There are frequent examples of callers telephoning more than 20 times; 50 calls, while rare, are not unknown.

The odd one really ought to see a shrink

Where 'acceptable variety' ends and 'madness' begins differs from one society to another, and from one time period to another.[1] In a small village the local 'daftee' may be a much-loved character, but in the large city the same person might well be the client of a clinical psychologist, a psychiatrist or a psychotherapist, or a client of a member of whichever other professional group has been allowed by society to claim responsibility for these matters.

By being able to pass over to 'professionals' the weird ones, a helpline can rid itself of the need to deal with the 'out-of-the-ordinary' characters in society. But should the helpline pass the odd one over to 'professionals' and, if so, in what circumstances?

In the eyes of many people, what used to be thought of as perfectly harmless oddities have become the sole province of those who require 10 years' university-level education and training. It is often difficult to accept the beneficial effects for society of these changes, particularly difficult for those who may fear that their 'acceptable variety' is in danger of being labelled 'sick'.

The suspicion which many people feel towards these professional groups has much evidence to support it. This suspicion does not just come from gay men and lesbians; evidence of systematic incarceration of excessive numbers of young black people in psychiatric hospitals provides another example.

It has taken over 100 years to get even part of the way to removing gay sex from the purview of such professionals. The failure of the church in Victorian times to squash all gay sex meant that the task was passed to medicine/psychiatry and to the law. The year 1967 saw a partial change in the law (concerning men).

At long last, in the 1980s the medical and psychiatric professions are beginning to take seriously some individual's mature preference for sexual relations with others of their own sex. This mature preference will finally be removed from the professional interest of these groups when those concerned stop seeking professional help for their 'homosexuality'.

If people suffer anguish as a result of society's hostility to gay men and lesbians, the best solution is to change the hostility, not create a new illness called 'homosexuality'. If the anguish has psychological or physical side-effects, then there may be a case for seeking medical assistance for those side-effects, but for them alone, not for 'homosexuality'.

Referring on

It seems universally accepted that no helpline should ever refer a caller to an outside professional without the prior consent of the caller (and of the professional). It is widely accepted, also, that even with consent no caller should ever be referred to a clinical psychologist, a psychiatrist or a psychotherapist unless that professional is fully aware of the nature and extent of the oppression of people like the caller.

The first of these prohibitions rests on a basic tenet of helpline work, namely that callers are in charge of their own lives. The second almost certainly means black psychiatrists (only) for callers to black helplines, and gay psychiatrists (only) for callers to gay helplines. Viewed rationally, this may be an unreasonable prohibition, but its roots are important and must not be dismissed lightly. A helpline would be placing in jeopardy its good-standing with its potential clientele if it were known to refer callers to members of professions with such poor reputations.

Professional assistance in cases where detailed counselling seems appropriate, however, is a different matter. Many helplines have trusted professional counsellors whom they use when necessary.

There is little criticism of these referrals when both caller and volunteer together agree that in order to deal with the problem more effectively they could benefit from bringing in an outsider with particular counselling skills. It is vital that the problem is not viewed as feelings of attraction to people of the caller's own sex. As part of this process the volunteer may need to acknowledge to the caller the limitations in his or her knowledge, experience and personal self-development, and may need to offer to work through his or her own limitations with a professional counsellor.

The legal and medical professions and the gay community

There are two other professions that might be expected to receive referrals from helplines – the legal and the (general) medical professions. How do helpline volunteers view members of these professions, and how do members of these professions regard helplines and the major focus of their work?

Many helplines make it clear that they are not qualified to give legal or medical advice. No doubt the legal and medical professions regard that position as being a 'responsible' one, but it does not solve problems about referrals. There are now specialist helplines dealing with legal matters and with medical matters associated with AIDS, and these are the recipients of many referred problems of a complex nature.

The legal profession

There is abundant evidence that high street provincial solicitors have little or no experience of dealing with, for example, 'cottaging' cases (explained below) or with lesbian-related child custody cases.[2] The effects on many lesbians of ill-informed assertions concerning lesbianism made by judges have already been considered. Perhaps an examination of the experiences of helplines over 'cottaging' cases may serve to explain something of the reluctance of gay helplines to refer callers to solicitors.

'Cottaging' is a slang term for the act of seeking casual sex in or near public lavatories. 'Cottage' is a gay male slang word for a public lavatory. Some activities concerning 'cottaging' are illegal, others are not.

One of the reasons why there is a startling disparity between the nature and quality of evidence in 'cottaging' cases and in other types of cases concerns the lack of expertise exhibited by solicitors. Too often the conduct of cases has owed more to feelings of disgust, guilt or embarrassment on the part of magistrates, the police, solicitors and the accused, than to a developed understanding of the law concerning the alleged offences.

For many of the offences which we group together as 'cottaging' matters, the accused has a right to elect for trial by jury rather than have the matter dealt with in a magistrates' court. The acquittal rate of jury-tried cottaging cases is much higher than the rates for almost all other types of alleged offence. The reason is that those with the courage to contest such charges before a jury know that they can present their case unfettered by the feelings of disgust, guilt or embarrassment which are present in a magistrates' court. Fortunately, the work over many years of Gay Legal Advice (GLAd) means that there is now a body of carefully documented evidence on the abuse of the legal system which occurs in many 'cottaging' cases.

'Go to see a solicitor' is advice which may subject the caller to pressure to plead guilty. This pressure owes more to the embarrassment of many solicitors who want to avoid being seen to defend such cases than to the facts of the case. Experts in this area assert that if trial by jury were a requirement for all these cases there would have been reform of the law on definitions of 'indecent', 'soliciting', and 'in public' long ago.

One might believe that the guilt feelings, which many people charged with 'cottaging' offences have, are sufficient in themselves to justify findings of 'guilty' of the offence as charged, whether or not in law they are guilty. To hold such a view is to claim that statutes should be interpreted according to the casual prejudices of the community at large – a view of law which flies in the face of the British legal system. Sadly, however, it would seem to be the view of many solicitors, and the view accepted by many 'cottagers' as well.

The solution to this problem may be to send a caller who requests legal assistance to a solicitor who had given callers, friends or acquaintances good service in the past on similar issues, and who is prepared to take seriously the aims of the helpline in trying to assist the alleged offender to have a better view of himself, and of his sexual disposition.

However, it may be important to ensure that the helpline's 'tame' solicitors do not acquire a reputation with magistrates for defending 'queers'. That may be just as damaging to a caller as an incompetent, embarrassed solicitor. It may also, incidentally, be damaging to the solicitor.[3]

The medical profession

When it comes to gay male sexual relationships, medical – as opposed to psychiatric – matters are raised only in the context of disorders where a means of transmission is through sexual acts, or in problems which concern physical sexual acts. There is no direct analogy between the failure of general practice solicitors to deal adequately with 'cottaging', and general practice medicine.[4]

The medical profession has long recognised that sexually transmitted diseases (STDs) are a specialism with which the general medical practitioner does not deal. Furthermore, there is a recognition of the unease felt by many who think they may have a sexually transmissable infection. Unlike other medical fields, where reference to a specialist must normally be made by a general practitioner, the general public may present themselves at a STD clinic without consulting a general practitioner first. In principle at least, these specialist clinics go some way towards maintaining anonymity by creating a nameless number system for patients; so that the call to consult the doctor is not a shout across the waiting room for 'Mr Macourt' but a call for 'number 258'.

Sadly, however, evidence on the relationships between STD clinics and their local and regional gay helplines reveals some distrust, antagonism and even occasional hostility. These negative reactions seem to occur when staff – particularly senior staff – have strong moralistic views about gay sex or where there is reluctance, for whatever reason, to co-operate with any part of the organised gay community on preventive health measures.

Alongside this must be placed some very useful co-operation between STD clinics and gay helplines in other areas; co-operation which has helped raise the level of awareness in the staff of STD clinics of the social problems faced by gay men and lesbians, and has helped raise the level of knowledge about sexually transmitted disorders within the gay world at large. The level of co-operation has increased since AIDS and HIV infection became an important issue, and even some hitherto hostile clinics have decided that they must co-operate with their local gay helpline.[5]

What about Eleanor – should she tell the police?

Stories of rape experiences are legion, stories of appalling handling by police and the courts are well known (though fewer new instances of *very* bad handling have emerged recently). Instances of women known to be lesbian being raped by men claiming 'all you need is a good fuck and that will turn you straight' are well known in lesbian circles.

These stories link the aggression and hostility of the outside world (of men) with being a woman who is a lesbian. Add poor handling by police and the courts and you have horror stories which (with reason) often seriously affect those women who hear them.

For example, take the case of Eleanor. Eleanor was just beginning to cope with her feelings for other women when she was assaulted by a man who failed to subdue her and ran off before sexual intercourse had occurred. She had been in contact with the helpline for a few months already and was beginning to enjoy attending women's support evenings even though she felt ill-educated and unsophisticated in that company. So as soon as she had recovered from the initial shock of the assault she contacted the helpline.

Why had *she* been attacked? Did the man know she was a

lesbian? Was it her fault that she was attacked? Will she ever feel safe again? Was she any longer a complete person?

With the help of women volunteers she was able to face bringing the matter to the attention of the police, and she was put in contact with the local Rape Crisis Centre.

Volunteers reminded her of their almost-universal view that poor treatment is meted out to known lesbians and gay men by the police and she was urged not to mention that she viewed herself as lesbian. It may be that attitudes among more senior officers (with notable exceptions) are less antagonistic to lesbians and gay men than attitudes of junior officers.

Volunteers were able to help her through the worst of her feelings and help her begin to feel human again. But it may take a very long time for her tender self-esteem to flower. The trauma of that assault may never fully disappear. However the helpline can help her recover from a sense of personal violation and disgust with herself and can help her understand her own feelings for other women.

The role of volunteers of the opposite sex

Sooner or later the male volunteers may be able to play a role in helping Eleanor too. Not directly, not overtly – but by being caring people who happen to be men, and by being around on the frequent occasions when Eleanor visits the helpline's offices they may help her to see that not all men are violators of women's bodies. They can also help the women volunteers help Eleanor, put into a wider context both her assault and her feelings for other women.[6]

There are many instances when volunteers of the opposite sex can be of particular assistance to callers, and other instances where they can be of general assistance.

Professional help for volunteers

One final matter concerning the use of referrals to professional advisers: few helplines yet arrange to have outside consultants available for volunteers (as opposed to callers), though many seem to actively recruit to the helpline those who have professional skills in the fields considered in this chapter.[7]

These volunteers are often used by other volunteers as sources of detailed information, but seem to be used less frequently as resources for the personal development of the volunteers. Perhaps more helplines should provide greater support from professionals for volunteers in their work and in their personal lives. This might well enhance the quality of the work done by the helplines.

'How do I meet other transvestites?'

Forty years ago Dr Alfred Kinsey and his team were condemned when their research appeared to show that sexual behaviour between men was a widespread phenomenon.[8] (Five years later a parallel research study made similar claims for sexual behaviour between women.) For men the Kinsey team asserted that more than one-third of adult men interviewed had had at least one voluntary sexual experience to orgasm with another adult man. The condemnation of Kinsey's work was loud and widespread.

The Kinsey team's studies are still the major sources of evidence on sexual activity; their data and their notion of a spectrum are both widely quoted and misquoted in discussions on sex. Society has managed to forget the enormity of the claim concerning the extent of some same-sex contact; 37 per cent seems to have been too great a figure to handle, but many people remember the figure of 5 per cent (those men whose sexual activity is largely or exclusively gay).

Kinsey and his team faced immense problems in carrying out their investigation; for example, in trying to devise a way of interviewing people which did not alert them to the moral views of the researcher. The group of researchers also found that society would not believe their findings, however well researched and presented. Helplines, too, find themselves with problems in presenting what they believe to be true about the world, in ways to which people will listen.

One instance of this difficulty is that although helplines deal with illegal matters frequently (as do all counselling agencies), they seem to have very few calls concerned with sexual activity between adults and children. This may be because most adult-child sexual activity is inside the family, and, whether inside the family or not, most is between men and girls, not between men and boys. However, many people still hold the mistaken belief that adult-child sex is closely allied to 'homosexuality'. For the gay world, and for gay helplines, the two are separate and distinct, and it would seem that they are seen as separate and distinct by those involved in adult-child sex, too.

Another instance where helplines have difficulty in presenting what they believe in ways to which people will listen concerns 'transvestites'. Although the vast majority of those who declare themselves to be transvestites claim to be heterosexual, and although many of them claim to be disgusted by anything to do with gay sex, nonetheless they form a sizeable proportion – anything from 5 per cent to 20 per cent – of calls to gay helplines.

Men's clothes and women's clothes

For 'transvestism' or 'cross-dressing' (dressing in the clothes of the opposite sex) to be an issue there must be rigid rules about what clothes are men's clothes and what clothes are women's clothes.[10]

Not only must there be rules but there must also be benefits. There must be inbuilt inequities between the status and treatment of men and women. For some people to believe that they have a need to cross-dress they must live in a society in which there are certain benefits in dressing in the clothes of one sex rather than the other.

If there were not rules about what clothes were men's and what were women's then no one would know – let alone notice – that someone had dressed in the clothes of the opposite sex. That may be an obvious statement, but in discussions about 'transvestism' it is surprisingly rarely said.

Even in a society where there are some differences between men's clothes and women's, but where there is some overlap, the decision of a man, say, to wear clothes more usually worn by women would arouse little comment, and would not bring with it feelings of guilt.

In some social groups in the UK there are rigid clothes rules, and in others the rules are less rigid, and in a few groups there seem to be virtually no rules at all. Jeans and a sweater can be worn both by young men and young women, without any comment. Twinset and pearls still look out of place on someone who, otherwise, looks male. But what is it to look male? Is it a beard and moustache, is it the absence of developed breasts, or is it other – less tangible and more socially related – attributes?

The 'butch dyke' on the motor-bike is as much of a stereotype (of a lesbian) as is the handbag-carrying 'queen' (of a gay man). Both are seen to be adopting some of the social attributes common to the opposite sex in the manner in which they dress. However, even in a dress some women may seem to be very 'masculine'; even in a leather jacket, jeans and workwear boots some men may seem to be very 'feminine'.

Whose needs?

Many people use the clothes they wear as a means of expressing something about the way they see themselves. But the opportunity to express something about oneself may be severely restricted by what is thought to be acceptable in the locality. For example, what is acceptable clothing in the student world of jeans and a sweater, or the world of the pop star, may not be acceptable in the world of the 50-year-old man in a mining village.

For many people, however, perhaps the social needs have got mixed up with sexual ones. Achieving some form of sexual arousal may be connected with wearing certain sorts of clothes. Usually we think of sexual arousal depending on the figure, the smile or the personality of the other person, but in certain clothes a figure may look more inviting, a smile more appealing or a personality more interesting.

So these are considerations when looking at questions about clothes, and from these we can deduce two reasons why some men need to dress in women's clothes: because they are making a statement about how constricting social life is, or they have a need to achieve sexual arousal.

It is only when people overstep the mark that their ways of achieving sexual arousal are thought of as odd or described as 'kinky'. But again the social groups in which people mix determine what is labelled 'kinky'. Jacket, trousers, underwear and cap all in leather, with studs and chains as adornment is acceptable – even obligatory – in some gay men's bars in London, but might be a less acceptable way of achieving sexual arousal at a barn dance in a Methodist Church Hall in rural Cumbria.

A third reason why some men need to dress in women's clothing may concern the man's view of the place of women. A man may feel that he (as a man) is obliged to control, command and direct, and he may see women as being demure, ineffective, disorganised, and free from having to dominate. To be free from having to be boss himself, he may feel that he must dress in women's clothes. Without women's clothes he thinks that he cannot feel that freedom.

There is a fourth reason, too, and it concerns the gay issue. In the eyes of many people, men dressing in women's clothes is associated with 'homosexuality' – and condemned along with it. But there is another side to this coin: Jim.

Jim and women's clothes

Jim is in his early twenties and has very limited horizons and experience. He lives in a large village and enjoys his weekly visit to the nearest large market town. Having found his way by accident into the (only, partly) gay bar there, he was picked up by a man who took him home, where the man dressed in women's clothing before having sex with him. Jim has been trying it himself ever since. He has never dared to return to the bar. He telephoned the helpline because it had been featured on television, and because he had these strange feelings for other men: 'I wear women's clothes, too. Where can I meet others like me?'

A careful conversation established that he believed that he was, somehow, required to wear women's clothes if he wanted to express his gay sexual desires. And, in some sense, what he was asking was nothing to do with clothes, but was really: 'I fancy other men, where can I meet others.'

Society's linking of 'homosexuality' and cross-dressing in order to condemn both had rebounded for Jim. He believed his willingness to dress in women's clothes was a mark in his favour when seeking help in meeting others who wanted gay sex.

But for the men who walked down this road thirty or forty years ago (before there was any chance of sorting that confusion out), cross-dressing has become their version of sex, and for many of them it goes along with a disgust for gay sex and for those who enjoy it.

To encourage or not

Many gay helplines find the subject of cross-dressing difficult. On the one hand a gay liberation view holds much sway, namely, that 'We should encourage "transvestites" to reject the oppression of society on them', 'We should encourage them to "come out" as "transvestites" and set up their own groups and helplines', and 'We should give as much help as we can.'

This presumes a category of people, 'transvestites', and so the 'be/do' debate (discussed on pages 34–39) had an analogy here. By encouraging people to think of themselves as 'transvestites', the helpline is stopping them thinking about themselves as complete individuals. Helplines claim to provide a safe and comfortable environment in which callers can think through their problems for themselves, an environment where gay relations are seen as equal to, not inferior to, straight relations. Few volunteers seem willing to deny transvestites any encouragement, but many will go no further than to inform callers of known meetings of transvestites when that information is specifically asked for.

The major alternative view to encouraging transvestites sees the social consequences of transvestism as contrary to a 'proper' understanding of women and men.

What about women?

Given the parallels between gay liberation and women's liberation, and given their common understanding of what it is to be human, many argue that no gay helpline should do anything which denies the equality of women with men.

It is argued that 'transvestism' must be rejected because it fails this test on several grounds. 'Transvestism' reinforces the inferior status of women, it reinforces the importance of certain traits which used to be thought to be womanly and others which were thought to be manly, and it denies the acceptability of same-sex relationships by emphasising sex differences.

Both of these views – to encourage, or to reject as contrary to women's interests – pressure gay helplines and make their treatment of cross-dressing a matter of much discord. Because of these pressures one view seems to get lost too easily.

Cross-dressing may be a harmless hobby. To see it as anything more is to encourage those who cross-dress to see it as something more, and to point out its anti-feminism to them may encourage them in that, too, as a reaction.

Helplines will continue to have widely different practices concerning cross-dressing. Perhaps no one approach is sufficient, perhaps there needs to be an approach to the young man, like Jim, who has got confused between cross-dressing and 'homosexuality', which is different from the approach to the middle-aged men who sit round transvestite groups trying to look demure and feminine, dressed in styles which often seem to owe a lot to the fashions of Marilyn Monroe and Dorothy Squires.

'If you want a good time why telephone us?'

Underneath all their questions, and behind all their anguish, most callers to gay helplines are seeking sexual satisfaction. To be acceptably accurate that sweeping assertion must be hedged about with qualifications such as 'alongside emotional and spiritual well-being'.

A general problem facing volunteers on all helplines, not just gay ones, is which should predominate: giving callers what they want, or what is good for them? That is not just about sex.

If one accepts that callers are seeking sexual satisfaction, ways in which helplines do, could or should provide that satisfaction need to be considered as should the bases on which callers take their decisions on these matters.

Put bluntly, sexual satisfaction could be provided by the volunteer (if of the appropriate sex) – acting as a sort of sex therapist, or prostitute. It could be provided by giving the caller lists of relevant names, contact addresses and telephone numbers.

Surrogates for sexual experience, which may carry with them elements of sexual satisfaction, could be provided by giving the caller access to sexually titilating reading or viewing material, or by providing a suitable aural environment, for example, by permitting the caller to masturbate while telephoning the helpline.

The issue of 'wankers' causes much anguish and many debates between volunteers. This section is primarily concerned with the matter of 'wanking calls', but first the other related matters must be considered.

'We are not a dating agency'

Gay helplines often respond to explicit requests for sexual partners with this response: 'We are not a dating agency.' A refusal to provide details of commercial dating agencies, may mask an objection to casual sex. Another view is that helplines are afraid of public objection if it were widely known that such information is provided.

A view of sexual relations which more usually underlies these refusals is an empowerment view. Many such services are thought to exploit their customers, financially and emotionally. Individuals should be assisted to reach a state of mind where they feel able to make friendships, and then the decision people take about whether those friendships develop into sexual liaisons or not is their own. So to provide them with access to agencies who could exploit them is held not to be in the caller's best interests.

A helpline may wish to assist individuals to achieve a state of personal maturity without wishing to impose any particular view about monogamy or about casual sex because these are seen as matters on which individuals must work out their own view. Volunteers see this as a reasonable approach which tries to prevent insecure persons from coming to excessive harm without molly-coddling them.

However, the issue of whether to provide access to dating agency services is far from settled within those helplines which see themselves primarily as a gay community information resource. Increasingly the view prevails that the helpline has no right to withhold information from a caller, unless that information is only available from the helpline. If information is available on, say, dating agencies, in newspapers and magazines – particularly perhaps if that information is available in journals aimed at a general audience, not merely a gay audience – then the helpline cannot refuse to pass it on.

The balance is struck – in a sense – between competing influences by (in some cases) refusing any information deemed to be sexist, racist, or anti-gay. These prohibitions are seen to be consistent with the view that all human beings are equal, and are responsible for their own actions. Any action on the part of a helpline which denies that view is unacceptable, whether it be condoning racism, or refusing adults access to sexual information about sex and sex-related facilities.

Sex as therapy

No manager of a helpline can place hand on heart and state with certainty that no volunteer has ever had sex with a caller. Helplines are subject to many pressures when agreeing their rules on this matter. First and foremost are considerations of exploitation of callers, second the response of the general public, third the response of the gay world and fourth faithfulness to a liberationist perspective.

As far as I know there has only been one gay helpline where sex was not barred between caller and volunteer. That helpline believed that by placing sexual taboos on the volunteer/caller relationship, such taboos were being reinforced in the lives of the callers.

Volunteers were trained not to exploit. This required a far higher level of training than is usual in helplines (or than is described in this book). It required a much deeper level of self-knowledge on the part of volunteers. Under all of these conditions there was no prohibition on consenting, non-exploitative sex. By the time it closed, the helpline concerned was one of the longest established, and had a very good record on these matters which was envied by many helplines which do operate prohibitions.

The public has varying expectations concerning gay organisations. It is clear that many people believe that all activity concerning the gay world is deplorable, and that – in particular and almost by definition – gay men cannot and do not act responsibly. Leaving aside this state of mind, which cannot be considered in a study such as this, there is another view about caring services in general which is widely held, and that is an expectation that no carer can expect to get personal gain out of caring.

Alongside this must be considered the view that it is very difficult to create a non-exploitative environment. It may be a grand ideal, but it is almost impossible to achieve.

Whatever rules a helpline has concerning sexual contacts with callers, however strongly it prohibits such contacts, the helpline will have a problem in the jealousy directed against its volunteers, and in particular its male volunteers.

Within the gay world accusations are sometimes made about male volunteers exploiting their position to procure for sexual purposes unsuspecting men who are not yet initiated into the ways of the gay male social scene.

There is some evidence that this view is beginning to wane in importance, but it is still frequently reported as the substance of male 'pub talk'. In a large conurbation, those volunteers who find this sort of conversation disquieting can remove themselves to a different social environment. For them this pub talk has little effect on morale, but in smaller centres where such separation is neither possible nor desirable it can be rather damaging and had, in some instances, been so damaging as to be a major contributory factor in the collapse of a helpline.

The jealousy which promotes the 'pub talk' can be seen as another manifestation of the self-hatred which many gay men feel. It is sad that it can be so damaging, but it may be a pointer to the future. Only in those places where such 'pub talk' has been reduced to an acceptable minimum can there be thought to be a social environment suitable into which new people may be introduced without damaging still further their self-image.

The grey areas

Returning to the theme of providing callers with sexual gratification we need to consider what constitutes sexual gratification. So far I have been considering overt physical sexual activity provided either by helpline volunteers or by people introduced by them explicitly for the purpose of sex. But if we extend the definition we find ourselves in the realm of helpline fund-raising discos!

It is worth noting that many helplines in small towns sponsor discos and other social events. Others sell *Gay Times, Gay Life* or *Gay Scotland* or act as distribution points for the *Pink Paper* or *Capital Gay*. Of course opponents of gay men and lesbians may try to present even these activities as the provision of opportunities for sexual gratification. But these helplines provide a caring service for their callers by providing a social environment which may be less aggressively sexual than the commercial one. They are also providing access to material about the gay world so that callers may feel more self-confident.

The 'wankers'

'Wanker' is the label given by helpline volunteers, in their internal conversations, to those men (this is an almost exclusively male phenomenon) who telephone helplines, are sexually aroused by conversing on sex-related themes, and who masturbate while holding the conversation with the helpline volunteer.[11] (As with many other issues dealt with in this book, this is not restricted to gay helplines.) How should helplines deal with these callers?

Some callers who are talking about their own gay feelings for the first time find that they become sexually aroused. Occasionally such a caller will acknowledge this arousal to the helpline volunteer. Such an acknowledgement is usually thought to be a sign of trust between caller and volunteer. Such callers are generally *not* thought of as 'wankers'.

Should helplines condone the activity of 'wankers' or should it be seen as an affront to the personal integrity of the volunteer? Should these men be encouraged to talk through their sexual frustrations with the volunteer?

Many women volunteers report themselves offended by having to listen to a man who is believed to be masturbating during the conversation. Some men are similarly offended. It is argued that the role of the volunteer is to be available for discussions of difficulties, however personal, but that the helpline is not available for cheap sexual thrills. Those who hold this view have indicated that they see the masturbatory activity of men while talking to women as a form of sexual abuse of women.

'Talk dirty to me' is a not uncommon request, and helplines have had to work out how to deal with the request. It seems that to try to engage the caller in conversation about his problems when he wants to masturbate achieves little other than an abruptly terminated call. Attempts to encourage callers to discuss problems after they have reached sexual climax appear to be more successful, though still unlikely, and at the cost of tying up a telephone line for anything up to 30 minutes before any useful (in this sense) conversation can take place.

Some volunteers argue that permitting the caller to masturbate (in the safe environment of a conversation with a helpline volunteer) may give the caller the confidence in the helpline to call again to discuss whatever difficulties he may be having. If this is the case, it is claimed, then permitting the 'wanker' to masturbate is justifiable. However, if permitting the masturbation merely encourages the caller to telephone for another 'wank' on another occasion – without any requirement to discuss problems – then this is seen as an abuse of the helpline.

For those who feel isolated from any possible sexual contact with other men, then 'wanking' calls may be the only way the caller can reduce his isolation. By gently attempting to ensure that the caller does not feel rejected by the helpline, it is claimed that it may be possible that callers will open up. As long as the caller is fully aware – as aware as words can make him, while he is masturbating – that the helpline is not to be abused, that empathy is available, and that he can talk as long as he needs to, then tolerating 'wankers' is seen as acceptable.

There is one tactic advocated by those unhappy with accepting 'wanking' calls. It is to make several abrupt changes in the topic of conversation (if it may be so called) – for example, suddenly changing from 'dirty talk' to something serious just as the caller is reaching sexual climax. They claim that it achieves some success, but at a price. The caller who does not pursue a conversation about his problem on that occasion is not likely to call back because his sexual climax was ruined.

AIDS and 'wankers'

In some major cities in the USA there are now established services where 'talking dirty' is encouraged. These services are designed specifically for those men who wish to avoid the gay scene through fear of AIDS and HIV infection. It is difficult to think of this development in the same light as the 'wankers' and it may be useful to consider the differences.[12]

Callers to the USA lines are motivated by a response to a particular phenomenon. They seek to have sexual pleasure without any risk of contracting AIDS or, for some, they wish to have sexual pleasure without endangering the health of others since they know that they are HIV positive or have been diagnosed as persons with AIDS. Clearly there is some justification for this development.

Callers to provincial helplines in the UK who wish to masturbate rarely have such cogent reasons for doing so, and when they do these reasons relate to isolation from any gay-related social environment.

Dealing with masturbatory calls is hard work. It can bring rewards to the volunteer when noticing progress in the caller's life, but this is very rare.

7 Improving Helplines

We need to assess the quality of helplines – helplines providing services and fulfilling functions which are not fulfilled adequately (if at all) by other agencies; and we need to assess the quality of work done by individual volunteers in providing appropriate and adequate assistance to each caller.

We must establish criteria for judging the quality of work done by helplines and that requires us to consider the functions which helplines fulfil through the services which they provide.

Then we need to examine whether any or all of these services could be provided by other agencies. In particular we need to consider the relationship between the work of general counselling helplines and the work of specialist helplines.

All this provides the backdrop for an answer to the question posed in the title : *How Can We Help You?* and an assessment of the future of helplines and in particular gay helplines.

What functions do helplines have?

There seem to be five types of service provision each of which fulfils an important function. The five are: to be a source of information; to be a neighbour; to be an entry point to a new world; to provide counselling and therapy; and to provide a focus for campaigning for equal rights.

Each of these needs to be examined separately even though there may be some overlap. Any alternative providers there may be for each service need to be considered. I shall try to distinguish, where possible, those elements which are singular to *gay* helplines and those which apply more generally.

To be a source of information

The most obvious service provided by helplines is that of being a community information and welfare resource. Many helplines are established for precisely that reason, and many of them are very successful at ensuring that they have an up-to-date record of the facilities available to their specialist audience.

A helpline established to assist those newly diagnosed with cancer needs to be able to provide information about welfare benefits which may be obtained and about facilities available for support, just as much as a gay helpline needs to have access to an up-to-date list of social venues for gay men and lesbians.

To be a neighbour

Another obvious service of a helpline is that of providing a friendly neighbour who is prepared to lend a listening ear. This is a form of social service for those who are socially isolated, analogous to that provided by a neighbour or relative who is prepared to have a chat or listen to a moan.

To be an entry point to a new world

While this service may have analogies elsewhere, this is primarily a service offered by those helplines concerned with groups who feel detached from the wider community. Where the feeling of detachment is great, those outside who want to become part of the groups may need a point of entry. For gay helplines this is particularly important.

The level of difficulty of entry to the gay world depends on a large number of factors. Intensity of sexual feeling for one's own sex, tightness of social control in one's own world, willingness to take risks, the degree of public visibility of the gay world, and the *apparent* ease of access are all relevant factors.

For some people entering the gay world is like stepping over a very low boundary fence between one field and another. For others the fence is higher, but it can be clambered over with care. But for others it is like trying to enter a forbidden garden which is surrounded by an extremely high wall. Access may only be gained through a hidden padlocked door.

The gay helpline, therefore, sometimes acts as the guiding hand (over the low fence), sometimes provides the step over the high fence, and sometimes acts as the doorkeeper who holds the key. Furthermore there may be occasions where it acts as the light in the window, attracting passers-by.

To provide counselling and therapy

Many helplines deliberately set out to provide therapy in the form of counselling: for those recently bereaved, for those who have been recently diagnosed with an apparently terminal illness, or for those in relationship difficulties. Other helplines find that they provide such a service whether they intend to or not.

Many gay helplines provide what amounts to a clinic for sexual and relationship therapy, operated over the telephone. In being available for discussions of problems concerning sexual activity or relationships, gay helplines are providing a service which no other volunteer agencies currently provide for gay men and lesbians.

To provide a focus for campaigning for equal rights

Many helplines provide a focus for raising people's awareness of issues on which action by local or central government is sought. In being prepared to participate in campaigning for equal rights a helpline will probably enhance its reputation among those in the groups it seeks to serve.

Often a helpline which is in touch with the community it serves and is aware of the importance of the issues involved will be in a better position than an overtly political organisation to gain access to the media or to public authorities.

When such access has been negotiated the helpline is able to use the opportunity to present arguments concerning the political issue in question, emphasising (where necessary) those dimensions which concern the efficacy of the counselling service it provides.

The interpreter

Each of the five services offered contains a common theme. The helpline is acting as an interpreter of one world to another – the big wide world and the special world of the group being served – often doing so through the eyes of the political activist.

As a community information resource the helpline is helping those it serves make sense of the world they live in, and is making them aware of a world in which they are special. As a neighbourhood listening ear the helpline is developing the values of a special world while taking account of the values of the big wide world.

In providing an entry service the helpline is most obviously being an interpreter. It is interpreting the special world to the caller who is coming from the big wide world. The helpline is interpreting it in ways which will encourage the caller to join it.

In providing relationship counselling and therapy a helpline is allowing callers to find out for themselves where they stand when facing conflicting values of the special world and the wider world, and assisting them to search for their own lifestyle. For example, a gay man may see this as a conflict between monogamy and hedonism. The helpline is acting as interpreter for the sets of values expressed by the two worlds, but doing it through the filter of one who wishes to empower.

In providing a focus for campaigning, the helpline is bringing the needs of the special world to the attention of the big wide world in a form which it believes the wider world will understand. Gay helplines often, in addition, bring campaigning issues to the attention of a gay world much of which does not want contact with the wider world, because it is comfortable within its ghetto.

Consider the analogy of the language translator. For an interpreter to be needed means that people are speaking different languages. If two people speaking different languages have a lot of contact with each other their knowledge of each other's language will improve, and so their own language may alter to adopt common words, phrases and grammatical constructions. As this process continues the need for an interpreter may diminish. Alternately they may decide that they want less and less to do with each other, so the role of interpreter becomes more important, and may even change into that of conciliator.

So it is with helplines acting as interpreters of special worlds and the wider world. Helplines interpret worlds to each other, worlds which may be growing further apart or worlds which are coming closer together. If the worlds grow too far apart helplines may be the only types of agency which can act in a conciliatory role; indeed they may be the only ones willing to conciliate. Helplines must be aware of the dynamics of change in and between the two worlds and make appropriate changes.

Who else could provide these services?

Are there alternative providers for each of the five services?

In most cases the *information service* could be taken on by a county library service, supplemented by a telephone inquiry service. However the political will to do so has to be found in order to ensure the provision of adequate resources.

Another alternative community information resource is 'word of mouth' around existing social facilities. However, this is no use to those who are isolated from existing facilities or who have yet to find an entry point to those facilities.

In the case of the information service, there are two additional problems for gay helplines. One is that many people who are afraid of their own feelings about sexuality, but who are able to pluck up the courage to contact a gay helpline, would not have the courage to seek out information in a public library.

The second is the additional pressure on a library service provided by those who are actually hostile to gay men and lesbians. The provision of information on gay and lesbian matters is politically contentious in some parts of the UK (in other areas it is not contentious because the local authority refuses to admit that there are any gay men or lesbians in its area).

This situation has not been aided by the pernicious section 28 of the Local Government Act 1988. It seems that section 28 does not affect the providing of information on gay and lesbian facilities.[1] However, there is evidence of some antagonists using the threat of an action under the section to deter library services from providing what little is currently provided.

Society is becoming increasingly complex. Long gone (if ever they existed) are the cosy villages with lots of caring neighbourliness. We no longer inhabit one 'neighbourhood', we all inhabit different ones for different dimensions of our lives: one for work, another for school, another for each of our interests, and (of course) one for where we live.

In one respect it is possible that the need for helplines to act as a neighbour is diminishing. Despite the efforts of racists and bigots, many socially outcast groups are becoming more integrated into society. So, for example, as the gay issue becomes a part of the experience of us all (whether oneself, one's family, friends or neighbours) and if there is a reduction of the antagonism heaped on gay men and lesbians, then this *neighbour* service might eventually be provided by the wider community.

However, there seems to be no obvious alternative service to act as an *entry point* (for the gay world, at least), except in a society which completely accepts same-sex relationships and where the boundary fence becomes invisible and people can cross and re-cross it at will. Over the last 30 years the boundary fence has been getting lower and lower, but the picture has become confused since the identification of AIDS and HIV infection.

Several helplines have indicated that there has been a drop in the number of male 'entry point' calls since mid-1984. Part of this drop is accounted for by the increasing visibility of the gay world – directly as a result of the publicity surrounding AIDS – and consequent ease of access without recourse to the good offices of a helpline. But another part of the drop, however, must be accounted for by the fear which many potential male 'new entrants' to the gay world have of becoming infected with HIV. The media have done them a disservice by claiming (incorrectly) that becoming infected is almost inevitable through involvement in the gay world.

In principle at least, other agencies could provide relationship *counselling and therapy*. Agencies specialising in relationship problems could deal with gay-related relationship problems, it is argued, and agencies specialising in problems relating to sexual performance and technique could provide sexual therapy. This argument is considered further later.

There are many instances of gay helplines taking a leading role in *campaigning* for the rights of gay men and lesbians. This function could be fulfilled by other organisations. However, the special position of a helpline as a 'caring agency' allows it forms of access sometimes denied to more overtly political groups.

Should counselling be handed over to generalist helplines?

Some people argue that generalist helplines (of which the Samaritans is the best known) are better qualified to deal with gay-related counselling problems because of their greater experience in a wide-range of personal problems and because counselling is their main function.

It is important to ensure, before addressing the merits of this case, that those advancing it are not seeking thereby to make the gay issue less visible ('If you advertise these things then, of course, they will appear to be important') – a problem which many gay activists encounter in a wide variety of spheres.

The argument goes like this: it should suffice to have specialist gay information networks and therefore counselling matters should be passed over to those with a general training in volunteer counselling. Gay helplines should fulfil those functions which require particular knowledge of the gay world and should leave counselling functions to those who specialise in counselling, even if they know little of the gay world.

This argument is attractive for two reasons. Firstly, many callers to helplines make choices before contacting a helpline. Callers may contact the Samaritans about gay matters when they are seeking counselling because they think of that agency as specialising in counselling.

It is argued that gay helplines should take advantage of this perception and concentrate their efforts on two primary functions, being an information resource and providing an entry point to the gay world. They would then be able to devote some of their energies to acquainting volunteers who work for generalist helplines with the problems associated with society's disapproval of 'homosexuality', so that they may take account of these problems in their counselling work.

The second reason why it is an attractive argument is that it would allow the expertise of volunteer counsellors on generalist helplines to be used more frequently, and thus more effectively, with gay callers – releasing the gay helplines from the necessity to train their volunteers to deal with counselling problems.

There are two counter-arguments, one about the nature of social oppression and the other about relationships between helplines founded on different bases. The underlying problem concerns the nature, extent and awareness of discrimination against women and gay men. If – but only if – there were detailed training for volunteers on generalist helplines on the forms which discrimination takes in society, and if – but only if – there were close, regular and detailed discussions between the two types of helpline, then could generalist helplines provide an alternative for the counselling currently provided by gay helplines.

There seems to be no desire on the part of most generalist helplines to attend to these matters. Many generalist helplines do not have a statement of principle about the equal validity of same – and opposite – sex relationships. This may be because such a statement would be controversial, or because of a desire to keep statements of principle to a minimum.[2]

Whatever the reason, the failure of many generalist helplines to accept such a statement of principle has profound consequences. Such a statement represents the least extreme position taken by gay helplines, so only when such a simple statement of principle is willingly adopted, and widely understood, will gay helplines feel confident that the counselling service they currently offer can be adequately covered by generalist counselling helplines.

Relationships between generalist helplines and gay helplines vary immensely. In many cases the relationships are good and an appropriate exchange of information and training takes place. In many other cases each helpline ignores the others. Sadly in some cases the relationships are inappropriate.

Three examples of inappropriate relationships will serve to demonstrate the variety:

- In one case every caller who mentions anything to do with the lesbian or gay issue is almost automatically referred to the gay helpline regardless of whether the reason for telephoning had anything to do with this issue.
- In another case the level of antagonism towards the gay helpline was so great that there was a consistent point-blank refusal to have any meeting at any level.
- In a third case all callers who raised the gay issue are almost automatically referred to one particular psychiatrist well known in the locality for his moral opposition to same-sex relationships.

Inevitably with widely diverse helplines there are bound to be extremes of relationships. However, the existence of extremes does not bode well for the transfer of counselling calls from one helpline to another.

It seems to be not just in relation to gay issues that generalist helplines have failed – if failure it be – but in relation to the issues which form the focus of many other specialist helplines (such as disability, common ethnic origin, etc.). These helplines would not have been necessary if their initiators had believed that the generalists were providing an adequate service. However, this may be more of a criticism of the nature of volunteer organisations rather than of generalist counselling helplines.

Similar arguments concerning transferring the counselling functions of gay helplines to generalist helplines can be extended to the transfer of particular counselling activities to specialist counselling helplines, for example marriage advisory services and child abuse helplines.

Five functions and nowhere to go

Three of the functions are, arguably, redundant because there are other agencies which could fulfil them if they would and if sufficient trust concerning both their ability and willingness could be built up.

The two other functions, an information resource and an entry point – remain to be fulfilled regardless. But these are the two functions involved in rapid changes in society, not least because of the impact of AIDS and HIV infection.

Assessing quality

Taking the notion of 'empowerment without exploitation' and translating it into the practice of volunteer and helpline allows certain basic statements of quality to be made.

The problems of judging what is good practice are immense. Without a previous body of tried and tested criteria to which to refer, any statements about quality are likely to be thought of as platitudes by some readers. Please bear with me. The statements I make must stand or fall on the following basis:

- whether they match up to the balance of influences incorporated in the notion of 'empowerment without exploitation' and
- whether they seem self-evident from the reader's experience of helplines (of whatever sort), experience which may have been gained through reading this book or through personal experience of telephoning a helpline or working on one

Characteristics of a good helpline

A good helpline is one

- which takes its work seriously, but which never allows its volunteers to become bored – or boring
- which is clear about why it wants to provide the service it offers, while never allowing its volunteers to thrust services down callers' throats
- where procedures are monitored in order to change and improve the service, but where volunteers do not find the monitoring intrusive because it is carried out sensitively and its purpose is agreed in advance
- where the volunteers enjoy each other's company, without allowing the helpline to become their only social circle

Characteristics of a bad helpline

A helpline is not discharging its responsibility to the community properly if it

- fails to operate at the time specified in its advertising
- permits people to join it and answer the telephone without training or assessment
- fails to update information files

But what of the individual volunteer? Volunteers are not giving enough of themselves to their work for the helpline if they

- fail to listen carefully to the caller's question
- put the telephone down during a conversation with a caller
- fail to turn up at the appointed time for a meeting arranged with a caller

The other side of the coin is that good helpline volunteers recognise why they want to be, and why they need to be, volunteers on a helpline. They take the work seriously but ensure that they build up enough self-confidence to be able to be naturally calm and friendly when answering the telephone or meeting a caller. They always see the caller as an individual, and not as another case – or bore – or chore. They know when it is time to stop being a volunteer, for a while, or altogether.

How can a good helpline be distinguished from a bad one?

A good helpline is not afraid to spell out what it sees its functions to be, and how it sees itself fulfilling them, because only if assumptions are made explicit can there be a degree of honesty between the helpline and the public. Without that degree of trust between helpline and public, honesty in dealing with callers cannot be assumed.

Therefore a good helpline has worked out, through *discussion* among all its volunteers, general guidelines and assistance for its volunteers on styles of work. It has achieved its own balance of the influences upon it. It has alerted the volunteers to a range of foreseeable difficulties, usually through a formal induction training programme and through an ongoing programme of in-service training. This process whereby volunteers discuss among themselves details of their work forms one part of a coherent *four-part monitoring programme* which good helplines undertake.

The second part of that programme involves keeping full *records* of all activities, with the immediate aim of assisting volunteers to deal more effectively with repeat callers and the longer-term aim of producing data which can be examined for trends. All sorts of trends may emerge from such an analysis, most of them requiring no great understanding of complex mathematics or statistics.

Examples of trends which may emerge include that certain types of call are becoming more frequent, that certain sorts of callers – women, or teenagers, perhaps – are more likely to call on one night rather than another, or at particular parts of the duty period. It may become clear that some volunteers have a noticeably higher, or noticeably lower, proportion of their callers calling the helpline again. (Where this is the case, over a period of a year, say, does the management of the helpline discuss the reasons for this with the volunteer?)

Each helpline will have identified the matter which particularly concern it, it will have established how best to empower callers in its own context, and it will have geared its monitoring programme appropriately.

The third part of a coherent monitoring programme involves taking account of reactions of the *public*. But where to start? Which public? The helpline checks its practices against the judgements of those in both the wider world and the special world to ensure that exploitation is understood and avoided, and empowerment maximised.

For some helplines part of this process involves listening to established groups which have some concern for the helpline. Perhaps there is a 'Friends of the Helpline' group who provide some of the funding for the helpline.

(Acting as a funding group often carries with it an implicit right to make criticisms of the helpline. However the helpline must still be responsible for its own activity. Volunteers must have the strength to stand up to funders who try to use control of the purse strings, in situations where they feel the donors are misguided.)

Some helplines hold open meetings at regular intervals at which a report of work done is presented and questions and criticisms sought. While it may be good discipline for a helpline, and particularly for its management, to go through such a procedure from time to time, this is essentially a self-monitoring process combined with a public relations exercise.

Listening to remarks made about the helpline in any social venues in which former callers are likely to meet is another source of public reaction, and is one way in which a helpline can come close to being accountable to some former callers. For gay helplines this involves listening to 'pub talk' since a high proportion of those men and women who are clients of gay pubs and clubs have used the services of a gay helpline at some time.

Other indications of approval by former callers include a steady flow of last year's callers seeking to become volunteers; frequent letters of thanks or return telephone calls of appreciation; and steadily increasing attendances at meetings of support groups set up for callers. Through monitoring these the helpline can become accountable to some former callers.

In a broader context some helplines are grant-aided from public funds, and most public authorities require evidence of proper use of resources. The evidence required may only be to satisfy them that the helpline employs proper book-keeping procedures, and maintain a basic record of the range of its activities. So a set of audited accounts and a statement about total numbers of calls with some elementary breakdown of callers by sex, age and marital status or location may satisfy a funding authorities. A poor helpline would not be able to provide even this minimal information, however the existence of such information is no guarantee of the quality of service provided.

Each helpline has its own means of monitoring public reaction, and if it does not – just as if it does not have any other part of a coherent monitoring programme – the question should be raised 'Is this helpline a good one?'

The fourth part of the programme involves other helplines of a similar type. Those helplines involved in a national or regional group find that the process of sharing experiences acts as a form of monitoring. In addition some groupings (for example in the gay helpline context, the FRIEND confederation) have moved towards a system of *peer review*, central monitoring by volunteers elected by fellow volunteers from all the helplines to undertake this work.

But how can I check?

So a good helpline has a monitoring programme which it uses to test its work against criteria of quality.

If the reader wishes to establish whether any particular helpline (gay or otherwise) is up to scratch, simply ask the management some of the questions outlined here. Before asking, however, satisfy yourself that the information is not just sought out of idle curiosity, and remember that helplines are volunteer organisations and dealing with your request for information may not (indeed should not?) have high priority.

The birth, life (and death?) of helplines

It would seem that there may be a pattern in the life-stories of helplines. First, some people recognise that an issue, whatever it is, requires action and they begin to do something about it. Then they realise that more people are affected by the issue than they realised, so they go about contacting them. Then they realise that they need to think more creatively about means of contact, that it needs the people affected by the issue to identify themselves and make the contact. And so a helpline is established.

Helplines *come into being* because people with idealism, vision and a desire to care see an issue which needs attention. Helplines *continue* because a steady flow of people who share the vision and the idealism are prepared to devote time and energy to caring and because the issue which forms the focus of their work has not gone away or been resolved. The volunteers settle down to develop a service, taking advice from others and learning to become a team of committed volunteers. They learn to help those coping with the issue to empower themselves and they help them avoid exploitation. Helplines continue because callers keep calling, the demand is always there.

Any helpline, which is a voluntary organisation, relies on the personal commitment of each volunteer to bind it together – nothing more, nothing less. Most volunteers fulfil their obligations to their helpline in addition to their occupation and domestic responsibilities. Few are free from other obligations.

Helplines *consolidate* because the volunteers are enjoying the work, and because the issue has still not gone away or been resolved. Most helplines work their way through any teething troubles. For example, it takes some helplines (particularly small ones) a long time to develop a coherent statement of purpose and this may lead to serious deficiencies in quality of service. It takes others (some of them quite large) a long time to realise the importance of having an adequate programme for monitoring the quality of the service offered.

Helplines *improve* when volunteers come in contact with people who renew the vision, who have new and fresh idealism and who have a desire to help more people and help them more effectively. These may be recruits, who must be trained well without them losing their vision or idealism. They may be volunteers on other helplines. Discussions with volunteers on other helplines renews vision, it rekindles idealism and improves standards. Or the people they come in contact with may be a fresh group of volunteers establishing a new helpline. (I have found that helping a new group of volunteers whose focus of interest is entirely different from one's own is a particularly valuable experience.)

Helplines *develop* when they have the enthusiastic support of the community they seek to serve. A helpline which is providing a worthwhile service is worth supporting, and a helpline which is worth supporting recognises that its service is appreciated and its volunteers work ever harder to ensure that they continue to deserve that enthusiastic support.

What happens next – and it may take only a few months or several years or it may seem like it is going to take forever – is that society at large becomes more aware of the issue and begins to deal with it. This may happen slowly at first, but then steadily and surely, as long as the pressure is kept up by campaigning organisations using evidence which the helpline can provide.

The death of helplines?

Helplines die in three circumstances.

- when society deals properly with the issues around which they exist. So the volunteers feel able to move on to other concerns, satisfied that their job has been well done – not just in the help they have offered individuals, but in persuading society to recognise and solve the problems around which the helpline was founded.
- when the community which the helpline seeks to serve ceases to appreciate the service it offers. This may happen when the service is inappropriate to the needs of the community, or because the helpline has devoted insufficient resources to explaining what its work is, and how important it is, in language which the community understands.
- when the environment around the community the helpline seeks to serve becomes so antagonistic – when the public hostility to the issue which the helpline exists to help with becomes too great – that volunteers and supporters can no longer sustain the helpline because they need to protect themselves and cannot afford to devote energy to protecting other people.

Can gay helplines die?

Gay helplines operate in a society which is in part supportive, in part hostile to their aims, but which is largely indifferent. Despite increasing recognition of the value of the work done by gay helplines from within social work, parts of the church, parts of the education service and even the police, indifference is ever present. Worse still, outright hostility is becoming rampant among a small but apparently powerful minority in society.

Gay helplines cannot be sure that there is going to be some progress on their issue sooner or later, and they have good reason to expect that life will get worse for gay men and lesbians before it gets better. Gay helpline volunteers have to cope with knowing that they (as part of the gay community) may have a fight for survival on their hands. But the last thing helplines need is antagonism from the society around them directed against the people they are trying to help, and even directed against the volunteers and the helplines themselves.

The last five years have seen gay helplines having to join the fight for the survival of the gay communities they seek to serve. Dramatic language? Not if you are contemplating what the media has done to your community over AIDS. Blame has been heaped by the media on you and your friends as you watch acquaintances and friends die – many of them people who were in the forefront of caring organisations within and outside the gay community.

Not dramatic language if you are faced with a government which gives in to its 'moral majority' wing, a wing that forced its hand so that local authorities are now prevented from 'intentionally promoting homosexuality'. Nobody seems to know what it means to 'intentionally promote', and nobody has attempted to define 'homosexuality' – except that it certainly does involve women and not just men, but the lack of adequate definitions doesn't seem to matter. Everyone plays safe. Nobody says anything about sex (except to condemn gay men or lesbians) just in case they might be contravening section 28. Even people with nothing to do with local government are being frightened into condemning gay men and lesbians, just in case they might be thought to be 'intentionally promoting homosexuality'.

What is next? More attacks, legislative, verbal and physical? What sort of society are we moving towards? *Not* a free market economy. A free market economy exists when all workers are free to develop themselves and be as enterprising as possible. A free market economy does not exist where access to employment is restricted to some because of the colour of their skin or their sex, or where workers can be sacked because of their choice of partner.

Yet the party which has development of the free market economy at the centre of its policies (which claims to support the abolition of constraints on workers and which has restricted the powers of trade unions) is the same party which is being held to ransom by a minority of its supporters, the so-called 'moral majority', which is neither a majority nor moral.[3]

Not a socialist society either. The struggle for socialism should be a struggle of all the oppressed against the oppressors. Like many others, gay men and lesbians are subjected to oppressive forces. So, in seeking to create a socialist society, the Labour party must fight to remove those oppressive forces as well as others if it is to remain true to socialism.

The Labour Party's record is only a little better than that of the

Tory Party. The last Labour government did little to improve the lot of gay men and lesbians and while it did include a pledge of full equality in its last election manifesto it has done little to follow that through since. In the House of Commons, the Labour Front Bench 'forgot' to oppose clause 28 until pressure from outside forced them to change their minds. In many of the local government councils it controls there is little support for gay men and lesbians. Until those borough party leaders controlled by the party who deny that there are any 'people of your sort' in 'our borough' are removed, it can have little credibility in the matter.

Parts of the new-look Labour Party, far from being a coalition of the oppressed (which might be able to build up a majority of votes), sometimes seem ready to become more extreme than the 'moral majority' wing in the Tory party they seek to replace.

The Democrats, SDP and Green Party come out of such an analysis well, but is this because they seem to have little chance of obtaining power (except perhaps in a coalition)? If they had power would they be any better?[4] Sometimes I doubt it.

The future for gay helplines?

Inevitably, trying to provide a gay helpline service in a hostile environment is not easy. The more hostile the environment the more difficult it is for volunteers to stand back from the hostility to assess their standards of service, and the more difficult it is for them to consider seriously any advice given to them from outside.

The degree of public hostility towards gay men and lesbians seems to vary markedly. The degree of impact which any hostility has on helpline volunteers also seems to vary markedly: from those helplines in large metropolitan areas which sometimes still claim that any talk of public hostility is outdated, to those helplines where a request from a local radio station for an interview is met with a refusal simply because no volunteer is prepared to risk the chance of violence or the possibility of being sacked from their job as a result of being interviewed.
environment is hostile is to help people feel strong enough to protect themselves and their communities. They must not frighten their callers with stories of hostility, but most continue to seek to empower them and help them avoid exploitation. Another role is to ensure that as many people as possible are aware of the impact of a hostile environment.

In a healthy society people can live and work to the fullest of their abilities in an environment in which they can overcome their anxieties about themselves. In the context of the work of gay helplines, this means overcoming anxieties about sexuality and relationships. We must all work for a society in which helplines and the whole community are on the same side, seeking to empower individuals, seeking to eradicate exploitation, seeking to alleviate anxiety, whatever group is the focus of a helpline's work – people who are newly disabled, black, bereaved, or gay and lesbian.

Good gay helplines deserve the support of the gay and lesbian community because helpline volunteers can only care for troubled gay men and lesbians if they know that they themselves are cared for and supported. One way to show helpline volunteers that their work is valued is to offer practical support – such as money and time – to enable helplines to help more lesbians and gay men and their families and friends.

Good gay helplines deserve the support of the whole community because they seek to ensure that people sort out their lives, their loves and their sexuality. If gay helplines did not exist, life would be more difficult for those people who are struggling to make sense of their sexual orientation, and for all those around them.

Notes

Introduction

1 For example the Council for Voluntary Service for Newcastle upon Tyne is in contact with 14 different volunteer telephone helplines (covering a wide range of specialist interests) within the city which has a population of under 300,000. *Telephone Counselling – List of Agencies Providing Counselling Services*, Newcastle CVS, Information Sheets, No. 24, 1988.
2 The figure of 80 represents a rounded average of the number listed in *Gay Times* in its monthly listing over the years 1987 and 1988. The publication of records of gay helplines is patchy and it is often difficult to interpret them since there are several instances of data referring to new callers only, or to calls where words were spoken only. The figure of 400,000 represents an estimate of the total number of telephone calls received by the helplines.
3 Pilot, Harbinger and Turning Points are names which have been used by these services. Pilot declares itself to be a 'service for homosexual relationships between persons of the same sex . . . a remedy is available to deal with the condition' (quoted from several different pieces of advertising material).
4 Weeks, J. *Sexuality and its Discontents: Meanings, Myths and Modern Sexualities*, Routledge and Kegan Paul, 1985, p.66.
5 *Gay Times*, monthly, publishes a list of helplines.
6 It would appear that, in important ways, the experiences of volunteers working for London gay helplines differ from those of volunteers working outside London. In part this reflects the differences between working in a metropolis, which has a very large and very public gay and lesbian population, and working in areas with apparently less supportive environments.

Chapter 1

1. A short history of the Samaritans is included in *Answers to Suicide*, Constable, 1978 (a volume presented to Chad Varah by the Samaritans on the 25th anniversary of their founding.
2. See for example Vining, R., *Training Samaritans*, The Samaritans, 1982 and Murgatroyd, S. 'Training for Crisis Counselling', *British Journal of Guidance and Counselling*, July 1983, vol 11 (2), pp.131–144.
3. Though there are signs that Dame Jill Knight MP and David Wilshire MP, with their direct attack on gay men and lesbian women – through their proposal which became section 28 of the 1988 Local Government Act – may have had a considerable effect on that debate within *gay* helplines, by ensuring that many volunteers recognised as important a political commitment to what they had regarded merely as a humanitarian concern.
4. Principle 1 of the Samaritans: 'The Samaritans are a fellowship of volunteers dedicated to the prevention of suicide', *Answers to suicide*, p.189.
5. See for example Wellings, K. 'Tracking Public Views on AIDS', *Health Education Journal*, 1988, 47(1), pp.34–36, and Jensen, L. *et al*, 'Attitudes towards homosexuality: a cross-cultural analysis of predictors', *Journal of Social Psychiatry*, Spring 1988. pp.47–57.
6. Anecdotal evidence of this type might lead to actions in the courts. However, a relevant instance is considered in Burton, P. 'The Enemy Within', *Gay Times*, August 1988 (119), pp.28–29.
7. A clear example of this sort of advice comes from the standard text recommended for Anglican clergy in training from the mid-1960s until the early 1980s, Waddams, H. *A New Introduction to Moral Theology*, SCM Press, 1964. Waddams advice was 'indulgence in homosexual practices . . . is morally wrong. Homosexuals should understand that they cannot physically satisfy their sexual cravings without moral blame. Indulgence in homosexual practices undermines [the 'homosexuals'] strength of character and often diminishes their artistic ability.' (rev. ed 1972, p.146–7) This does not represent a conservative position. SCM Press has long had a reputation for publishing material at the liberal end of the Christian spectrum.
8. An early statement for change was made in Righton, P. (ed) *Counselling Homosexuals: A Study of Personal Needs and Public Attitudes*, Bedford Square Press/NCSS, 1973.

9 And, of course, there are many professional counsellors who proudly acknowledge their personal identification with the gay and lesbian communities. An important service, funded by the London Boroughs Grants Scheme, is that run by PACE (the Project for Advice, Counselling and Education) at the London Lesbian and Gay Centre, 67–69, Cowcross Street, London, EC1M 6BP.
10 For details of the teachings of gay liberation see: *Manifesto*, Gay Liberation Front, 1971; Altman, D. *Homosexual Oppression and Liberation*, Oughterbridge and Lazard, 1971; Weinberg, G. *Society and the Healthy Homosexual*, St Martin's Press, 1972; and *Psychiatry and the Homosexual*, Gay Information, 1973. For an outline of the British gay liberation movement see Fernbach, D. *The Rise and Fall of GLF*, London School of Economics Gay Culture Society, 1973 and Walter, A. (ed) *Come Together: the Years of Gay Liberation 1970–73*, GMP, 1980. For a useful critique of these teachings see Weeks, J. *Sexuality and its Discontents*, Routledge and Kegan Paul, 1985 particularly Chapter 8, pp.198–210 and for reminiscences of the period see Birch, K. 'A Community of Interests' in B. Cant and S. Hemmings (eds) *Radical Records: Thirty Years of Lesbian and Gay History*, Routledge, 1988, pp.51–59.
11 See for example Cant, B. 'Normal Channels' in Cant and Hemmings, *Radical Records*, pp.206–221.
12 The 1967 Act did not reflect an acceptance of male same-sex acts, rather the method and extent of control was refined. Both men involved in the sexual activity must be over 21, the activity must be in private (with a curiously restrictive understanding of privacy), neither must be a member of the armed services, members of the merchant navy are excluded in certain circumstances and when passed the Act only applied to England and Wales. For fuller accounts of its limitations see Sturgess, B. *No offence: the case for homosexual equality at law*, CHE, SMG & USFI, 1975; Crane, P. *Gays and the Law*, Pluto Press, 1982 and Warner, N. *Parliament and the Law* in B. Galloway (ed) *Prejudice and Pride: Discrimination Against Gay People in Modern Britain*, 1983, Chapter 5, pp.78–101.
13 Weeks, J. *Coming Out: Homosexual Politics in Britain from the Nineteenth Century to the Present*, Quarter, 1977, p.215. By 1977 the National Organiser of FRIEND (as the Chair of the National Committee is known) had ceased to sit of right on the CHE Executive Committee, and the FRIEND newsletter had ceased describing itself as the 'befriending organisation of CHE' as it had hitherto.

14 Weeks, *Coming Out*, p.169, and Horsfall, A. 'Battling for Wolfenden' in Cant and Hemmings, *Radical Records*, pp.15–33. I am grateful to the directors of the Hall Carpenter Archive (when that archive was located at the London Lesbian and Gay Centre, 67–69 Cowcross Street, London, EC1M 6BP) for their assistance in providing information on the early days of the Homosexual Law Reform Society and the Albany Trust, and other matters.

15 Weeks, *Coming Out*, p.216 and *Gay News*, 9 May 1974 (46) pp.1 & 4, and *Gay News*, 15 January 1976 (86) p.10. In 1985 it was announced that Icebreakers no longer saw itself as a telephone helpline. *Capital Gay*, 20 September (210) 1985.

16 Weeks, *Coming Out*, p.218–9 and *Gay News* 14 March 1974 (42), p.1, and *Gay News*, 23 May 1974 (47), p.5. London Lesbian and Gay Switchboard operates a 24-hour service on 01–837 7324.

17 For an account of the history of *Gay News* see Hanscombe, G.E. and Lumsden, A. *Title Fight: the Battle for Gay News*, Brilliance Books, 1983. There were 35 gay helplines listed in the *Gay News Gay Guide* March/April 1976, a supplement to *Gay News*, (90, 91 & 92).

18 The first Lesbian Line, in London, began operation on 23 Sept 1977, *Gay News*, 7 Sept 1978 (150), p.7.

19 Watney, S. *Policing Desire: Pornography, AIDS and the Media*, Methuen, 1987 and Vass, A.A. *AIDS, A Plague in Us – A Social Perspective*, Venus Academica, 1986. A weekly column on AIDS which includes comments on press coverage began in *Capital Gay* on 27 July 1984 (154) under the authorship of Julian Meldrum until 25 July 1986 (252). It was taken over by Tony Whitehead on 15 August 1986 (255). A column entitled 'Mediawatch' which covers all matters in the press of concern to gay men and lesbians, not just AIDS, has been running in *Gay Times* for nearly five years. An excellent interpretation of the mass hysteria is given in 'Sex as Fear and Loathing: the example of AIDS', *Sexuality and its Discontents*, 1985, pp.44–53.

20 Homophobia is a concept developed in 1972 in Weinberg, *Society and the Healthy Homosexual*.

21 Vass, *AIDS. A Plague in Us*, p.137. Rev Greg Richards, who died on 31 Jan 1985, was not the first Anglican clergyman to die as a result of AIDS in England, but the press failed to find out about the first one. Julian Meldrum, reviewing the press coverage in *Captial Gay*, 8 Feb 1985, (178), commented: 'Richards died as the innocent victim of an accidental encounter with a virus. A virus that has no mind, no moral status. His reputation, however, was *murdered* [his

emphasis] . . . I am glad he didn't live to see it. Ironically, had he lived, the law of libel would have protected him.' (p.12)
This book is dedicated to the memory of one of the author's close friends, Frank Wilson, who was an intimate of Greg Richards. Frank died three months later on 1 May 1985.
22 See Altman, D. *Aids and the New Puritanism*, Pluto, 1986; Watney, S. 'Gay Rights in Britain and the USA', *Gay Times*, February 1988 (113), pp.37–39.
23 The Terrence Higgins Trust was founded in 1982 (*Capital Gay* (71), 26 Nov 1982).
24 See Orton, S. and Samuels, J. 'What We Have Learned from Researching AIDS', *Journal of the Market Research Society*, January 1988, 30(1), pp.3–34, and Wober, J.M. *Evaluating the Broadcast Campaign on AIDS*, Independent Broadcasting Authority, 1987. The advertising campaign was denounced by the press officer of London Lesbian and Gay Switchboard as 'irrelevant to gay men' in *Gay Times*, March 1987 (102), p.6.
25 The Labour Party, the Liberal Party, the Social Democratic Party, the Communist Party, Plaid Cymru, the Scottish National Party and the Alliance Party of Northern Ireland all contain commitments to equality which (implicity or explicity) included gay men and lesbian women.
26 Chris Smith came out at an anti-discrimination demonstration at Rugby on 10 November 1984. He was first elected in 1983 before he came out.
27 For good reviews see Kent-Baguley, P. 'One Too Many', *Youth and Policy*, Spring 1988 (24) pp.1–7, and Roelofs, S. 'Clause 28' in *Spare Rib*, April 1988 (189) pp.38–39.
28 Advice given by Michael Barnes QC to the Association of London Authorities as reported in *Gay Times*, May 1988 (116) p.7. Also see *Section 28: What Does It Mean for the Voluntary Sector?*, NCVO, 1988.
29 The atmosphere during the Synod debate and later developments are discussed in Leech, Rev. K. 'Crisis for Gays in Church of England', *Christian Century*, 20–27 July 1988, pp.678–9.
30 For example, the Bishop of Durham, in an address to his Diocesan Synod, 21 May 1988: 'Homosexuality is, for a limited but significant number of people, normal and we [the Church] have not yet come to terms with this . . . I will not enquire into the private practices and life-style of homosexual priests and ordinands more deeply than I would into the private practices and life-style of all other priests and ordinands . . .'

31 For an account of the matter see Macourt, M. 'Dealing with dishonour in the Church', *The Pink Paper*, 25 August 1988 (39), p.7. The author, a member of the Executive Committee of the Lesbian and Gay Christian Movement, has responsibility for the Movement's defence of the action.
32 See reports on the Pride March 1988 in London in *Capital Gay*, 1 July 1988 (349), p.1, and on the national demonstrations against clause 28 in Manchester in *Capital Gay*, 26 February 1988 (331), pp.10–11 and in London *Capital Gay*, 6 May 1988 (341), p.1.

Chapter 2

1 Since this is not a research monograph I have not attempted to reproduce detailed statistical evidence in support of my claims here and elsewhere concerning either the frequency of different types of calls or the relative proportions with which certain views are held by helpline volunteers. I am grateful to those helplines which have allowed me access to their detailed records and to those volunteers with whom I have had discussions. Published material on the work of helplines includes Halfpenny, P. and Cotterill, J. 'Who calls FRIEND?', *British Journal of Guidance and Counselling*, May 1986 14(2), pp.154–167 on the work of Manchester FRIEND May to July 1981; Conn, P. (National Organiser of FRIEND 1984–88), 'Profile of a Gay Help Agency', *Counselling*, August 1985 (53), pp.19–23; and Griffith, R.K. 'The Changing Pattern of Calls to an AIDS Advice Line'. *Health Education Journal*, 1988 47(1) pp.3–6 reviewing calls to Birmingham AIDSLINE January to July 1987. In order to respect the assistance I have received from volunteers in many helplines, the names in the examples used in this book have been changed, as have some of the details in certain instances where it might otherwise be possible to recognise the people concerned.
2 The British Association for Counselling Code of Practice states: 'Counsellors treat with confidence personal information about clients, whether obtained directly or indirectly by inference . . . "Treating with confidence" means not revealing any of the [personal information] to any person or through any public medium, except to those to whom the counsellor owes accountability for his/her counselling work . . . or on whom the counsellor relies for support and supervision.' See also Bond,T. 'Confidentiality', *Counselling*, November 1988 (66), pp.3–8.
3 An exception is *Changing the World: A London Charter for Gay*

and Lesbian Rights, Greater London Council, 1985, but the Greater London Council was abolished before many of the recommendations could be implemented. See also Davies, P. 'Local Boroughs – the Battle Goes On' *Captial Gay*, 18 August 1987 (307), pp.12–13. For further comments see Greasley, P. *Gay Men at Work*, Lesbian and Gay Employment Rights (LAGER), 1986.

Chapter 3

1. A useful review which raises many questions concerning the 'be/do' debate is King, D. 'Condition, Orientation, Role or False Consciousness?: Models of Homosexuality and Transsexualism', *The Sociological Review*, Feb 1984, pp.38–56.
2. Plummer, K. *Sexual Stigma: an Interactionist Account*, Routledge and Kegan Paul, 1975, Chs 3 & 7. An excellent spoof of the causes debate was produced in wall poster form in Wakeman, A. *Causes of Heterosexuality*, Gay Sweatshop, 1975.
3. Kitzinger, C. *The Social Construction of Lesbianism*, Sage, 1987.
4. Macourt, M.P.A.(ed) *Towards a Theology of Gay Liberation*, SCM Press, 1977. Another useful source is Boswell, J. *Christianity, Social Tolerance and Homosexuality*, University of Chicago Press, Chicago, Illinois, 1981.
5. There are several lesbian and gay Christian groups, the best known of which is the (ecumenical) Lesbian and Gay Christian Movement, which was founded in April 1976 and which runs its own counselling service. Others include Quest (for Roman Catholic men), Friends Homosexual Fellowship (Religious Society of Friends, Quakers) and the Catholic Lesbian Sisterhood (for Roman Catholic women). There are also several branches of the Universal Fellowship of Metropolitan Community Churches, a gay-and-lesbian-orientated church based in the USA.
6. The authoritative studies on this subject are Ford, C.S. and Beach, F. *Patterns of Sexual Behaviour*, Harper, New York, 1951 and Churchill, W. *Homosexual Behaviour among Males: A Cross-cultural and Cross-species Investigation*, Hawthorn Books, New York, 1967.
7. Difficulties abound in making this calculation, including problems of definition, comparing data from different sources, non-existent joint distributions and groupings which are insufficiently specific. Sources include *General Household Survey Annual Reports*, HMSO and reports of the *Census of Population for 1981*, HMSO.
8. Kinsey, A.C., Pomeroy, W.B. and Martin, C.E. *Sexual*

Behaviour in the Human Male, Saunders, Philadelphia, Pennsylvania, 1948 'Concerning matters of sexual behaviour a great deal of thinking . . . stems from the assumption that there are persons who are "heterosexual" and persons who are "homosexual" . . . it is implied that every individual is innately – inherently – either heterosexual or homosexual.' (pp.636–637)
'The histories which have been available in the present study make it apparent that the heterosexuality or homosexuality of many individuals is not an all-or-none proposition . . . Males do not represent two discrete populations, heterosexual or homosexual.' (pp.638–639)
'While emphasising the continuity of the gradations between exclusively heterosexual and exclusively homosexual histories, it has seemed desirable to develop some sort of classification which could be based on the relative amounts of heterosexual and of homosexual experience or response in each history.' (p.639). The classification, later called a rating scale, is the oft-quoted Kinsey scale. A companion volume containing data for women is Kinsey, A.C., Pomeroy, W.B., Martin, C.E. and Gebhard, P.H. *Sexual Behaviour in the Human Female*, Saunders, Philadelphia, Pennsylvania, 1953.

9   Consistently throughout 1987 and 1988 60–65 per cent of those reported as being HIV positive have been reported from the four Thames Health regions (covering Greater London and the Home Counties), and these regions contain 73–77 per cent of all diagnosed AIDS cases. Those regions contain approxiamately 25 per cent of the population of England and Wales (*Weekly Communicable Disease Reports* of the Public Health Laboratory Service).

10 However there have been many good books publishe . on the subject including: Altman, *Aids and the New Puritanism*; Fitzpatrick, M. and Milligan, D. *The Truth about the Aids Panic*, Junius, 1987; Richardson, D. *Women and the AIDS Crisis*, Pandora, 1987; Tatchell, P. *AIDS: A Guide to Survival*, GMP, 1986; McMullen, R. *Living with HIV in Self and Others*, GMP, 1988; and Aggleton, P. and Homans, H. (eds) *Social Aspects of AIDS*, Falmer, 1988. A fine collection of short stories with AIDS and HIV infection as their common theme is: Mars-Jones, A. and White, E. *The Darker Proof: Stories from a Crisis*, Faber & Faber, 1987.

11 However the formal evidence for this assertion is limited, see Coxon, A.P.M. *Homosexual Sexual Behaviour*, Social Research Unit, University College, Cardiff, Working Paper No.4, 1986, p.4. 'It is astonishing that there is little reliable

information . . . about even such basic facts as what proportion of gay men engage in high-risk behaviours.' and see footnote Ch.6, p.136, 1.2.
12 The proportion of those newly-reported HIV – who are known to be gay or bisexual men has declined from 73 per cent to 50 per cent between mid-1987 and mid-1988. (*Weekly Communicable Disease Reports* of the Public Health Laboratory Service).
13 Useful material on the counselling of people with AIDS or HIV infection is contained in Kirkpatrick, B. *AIDS: Sharing the Pain – Pastoral Guidelines*, Darton, Longman and Todd, 1988; in Spence, C. *AIDS: Time to Reclaim our Power*, Lifestory, 1986; in Miller, D. 'Counselling', *British Medical Journal*, 27.6.1987 (294) pp.1671–1674; and in Bor, R,. Miller, R. and Perry L. 'AIDS Counselling: Clinical Application and Development of Services', *British Journal of Guidance and Counselling*, January 1988 16(1), pp.11–20.
14 See Baker, J.R. 'On the Frontline', *Gay Times*, January 1988, (112) pp.44–47.
15 I am grateful to those involved in US gay helplines who have offered me observations on this and other matters.
16 Lambda, the greek letter l (λ) – for Lesbos, the Aegean island on which lived Sappho and her women – was a recognised symbol of gay rights organisations in the 1970s.
17 After several attempts to found such an organisation the present Gay Business Association was founded in 1984.

Chapter 4

1 Both FRIEND and London Lesbian and Gay Switchboard (LLGS) have produced details of programmes for selection and training of volunteers. See, from FRIEND: *Befrienders Kit*, various editions since 1977, and Silvester, K. *Recruitment and Training Guide* 1986, and from LLGS *Agreed Procedures*, various editions since 1979. A former national organiser of FRIEND also compiled two very useful short handbooks: Conn, P. *Setting up Handbook*, National FRIEND, 1986 and Conn, P. *Service Handbook*, National FRIEND, 1987.
2 The effect of training on the trainees has been noted in Walker, L.G. and Baird P. 'Marriage Guidance Training and the Trainee's Own Marriage', *British Journal of Guidance and Counselling*, May 1988 16(2) pp.176–189 and see footnote 2, ch.1.
3 From time to time, helplines find themselves coping with one unfortunate side-effect of the lack of public recognition

for their work. There are no effective sanctions available against charlatans moving in on gay helpline activity. There are still those who for purely selfish reasons present themselves as a new gay helpline, advertising their service wherever they can and reaping the 'benefits' in terms of new sexual conquests from among those who seek their services. There are also some new (genuine) helplines who begin operation without any adequate training and without any understanding of the enormity of the undertaking upon which they are embarking. There is no immediate control which established helplines can exercise on these two sorts of operation.

4   I can find no published information on acceptance rates for Samaritans, but this range has been confirmed by two Samaritans branch directors.
5   Charity registration number 296300.
6   The National Association of Gay Switchboards was formally founded at the 4th Annual Gay Switchboard Conference. London Gay Switchboard joined the association in 1981.
7   See Lyttle, J. 'The Reincarnation of London [Lesbian and Gay] Switchboard', *Gay News*, (35) 17 Jan 1985, pp.18, 19, 30. and Power, L. 'Voices in My Ear' in Cant and Hemmings, *Radical Records*, pp.142–154.
    See note 3, Introduction.
8   The latest – another arson attack on the London Lesbian and Gay Centre – was reported in *Capital Gay*, 12 August 1988 (355), p.1.

Chapter 5

1   Cramer, D. 'Gay Parents and Their Children: a Review of Research and Practical Implications', *Journal of Counselling and Development*, April 1986, 64(8), pp.504–507.
2   The Government announced its immediate support for the Wilshire/Knight clause 28, despite having opposed a similar move by Lord Halsbury only 12 months earlier.
3   Many cases studies are detailed in Greasley, *Gay Men at Work*. Lesbian and Gay Employment Rights (LAGER) has a commendable record in advising individuals and in ensuring that cases of discrimination are raised in the gay press.
4   See Barratt, M. and Harne, L. (eds for the Rights of Women Lesbian Custody Group), *Lesbian Mothers' Legal Handbook*, The Women's Press, 1986, pp.105–137; also Hanscombe, G.E. and Forster, J. (eds) *Rocking the Cradle: Lesbian Mothers – a Challenge in Family Living*, Sheba Feminist Publishers, 1982,

Richardson, D. 'Lesbian Mothers' in Hart, J. and Richardson, D. *The Theory and Practice of Homosexuality*, Routledge and Kegan Paul, pp.149–159, and Allen, S. and Harne, L. 'Lesbian Mothers: the Fight for Child Custody' in Cant and Hemmings, *Radical Records*, pp.181–194.

5 However, a useful survey is reported in Barratt and Harne, *Lesbian Mothers' Legal Handbook*, pp.138–170. Cases are reported frequently in the gay press, e.g. a report of a lesbian losing her 7-year-old son to his father six years after getting custody in the divorce, in *Gay Times*, August 1988 (119) p.7. See also McLeod, E. 'What Difference Does It Make – Should Homosexual Fathers be Given Custody?' *Social Work Today*, 12 March 1984 15(27), pp.12–13.

6 See Barratt and Harne, *Lesbian Mothers' Legal Handbook*, ch.3 'Finding and Coping with Your Solicitor', pp.33–39 and ch.4 'Out of Court Strategies', pp.40–45.

7 A useful comment on the study of gay and lesbian history is Dollimore, J. 'A History of Some Importance', *Gay Times*, August 1988 (119), pp.44–45.

8 Useful comments are contained in Poverny, L.M. and Finch, W.A. 'Gay and Lesbian Domestic Partnerships: Expanding the Definition of Family' *Social Casework*, February 1988, 69(2), pp.116–121.

9 See Shiers, J. 'One Step to Heaven?' in Cant and Hemmings, *Radical Records*, pp.248–258.

10 See Greig, N. 'Building Bridges – the Status and Role of Gay Theatre', *Gay Times*, December 1985/January 1986 (88), pp.74–76.

11 The Hall-Carpenter Archive presented itself thus: 'For many centuries history has made no acknowledgement other than a censorious or a patronising nod of the head in our [gay men and lesbians] direction. The lives and ideas and feelings of many a million brothers and sisters died with them. The Hall-Carpenter Archive is making this a thing of the past. It is dedicated to . . . every element of lesbian and gay history . . . taking pride in our history.' *Hall-Carpenter News*, June 1985.

12 Babuscio, J. *We Speak for Ourselves: The Experiences of Gay Men and Lesbians*, SPCK, 1988 (rev.ed). Chapter 7, 'Coming Together' contains an excellent account of the nature and diversity of the gay scene (pp.113–127). Additional useful remarks may be found in Brayne, A. 'The Big City Ghetto', *Gay Times*, January 1985 (77) pp.36–37.

13 I am grateful to the group concerned for the opportunity to participate as a castaway in Gay Desert Island Discs.

14 Auerback, S. and Moser, C. 'Groups for the wives of gay and bisexual men', *Social Work*, July/August 1987 32(4), pp.321–324.; Thorneycroft, B. Weeks, J. and Sreeves M. 'The Liberation of Affection' in Cant and Hemmings, *Radical Records*, pp.155–168; and Plummer, K. *Documents of Life*, George Allen and Unwin, 1983.
15 An early positive contribution to the issue of gay teenagers was a pamphlet produced by Birmingham Gay Liberation Front, *Growing up Homosexual*, 1973. The National Gay Federation (Ireland) produced a useful discussion document, *A Youth Group for Gay Adolescents*, 1979 and the Joint Council for Gay Teenagers produced *I Know What I Am: Gay Teenagers and the Law*, 1980 and published a collection of personal histories, Burbidge, M. and Walters, J. *Breaking the Silence: Gay Teenagers Speak for Themselves*, 1981. The London Gay Teenage Group published four reports: Trenchard, L. and Warren, H. *Something to Tell You*, 1984; Trenchard, L. *Talking about Young Lesbians*, 1984; Warren, H. *Talking about School*, 1984; and Trenchard, L. and Warren, H. *Talking about Youth Work*, 1985. See also Heathfield, M. 'The Youth Work Response to Lesbian and Gay Youth', *Youth and Policy*, Winter 1987/88 (23), pp.19–22.
16 The teenager group concerned compiled and published two useful documents in its early years: *Gay Teenagers Come Out, Come Out, Wherever You Are*, 1981 and a report on its first four years, *Tyneside Gay Teenagers' Group 1980-84*.

Chapter 6

1 See for example Szasz, T.S. *The Myth of Mental Illness*, Harper and Row, 1974 (rev.ed.) and Brown, P. (ed) *Radical Psychology*, Harper & Row, 1973.
2 Three useful sources provided evidence for this section – Galloway, B. 'The Police and the Courts' in Galloway, *Prejudice and Pride*, pp.102–124; Crane, P. *Gays and the Law*, Pluto Press, 1982 and Cohen S. (ed for Manchester Law Centre) *Law and Sexuality*, Grass Roots Books, 1978, particularly pp.116–124. Useful comments on the importance of 'cottaging' to some gay men can be found in Burton, P. 'The Cottaging Taboo', *Gay Times*, February 1985 (78), pp.36–39.
3 Many gay men see a solicitor only (if at all) to make wills. The Gay Bereavement Project and GLAD (Gay Legal Advice) both confirm that partners make wills to avoid complications with hostile families.

4 But see Marshall, J. 'The Medical Profession' in Galloway, *Prejudice and Pride*, pp.165–193.
5 The co-operation which there has been concerning AIDS and HIV infection, while in marked contrast to government support for the Wilshire/Knight section 28, leaves a great deal to be desired. It is patchy. In large metropolitan areas many health authorities seem to be very concerned to involve gay helplines in their work. In other areas, however, it would seem that the fear of being associated with known 'homosexuals' is too great for many health authorities and so co-operation is often non-existent, even under pressure from the gay helplines.
6 Many gay male volunteers feel that they have reason to fear the police and are antagonistic towards their helpline having any involvement with them. Despite very many instances of police humiliation of gay men there are also a few instances of police co-operation with gay helplines. Talks to recruits at police training colleges and training exercises for the Vice Squad are uncommon but not unknown. Reports of police antagonism appear in almost every issue of gay newspapers. For a review of the attitudes of the police in London see Davies, P. 'What's Going On 'Ere Then? A Special Report on the Metropolitan Police', *Capital Gay*, 8 January 1988 (324), pp.10–11. The work of the police monitoring groups in London, Gay London Policing Group (GALOP) and Lesbian Policing Project (LESPOP) is noteworthy.
7 See Conn, P. *Services Handbook*, pp.28–29.
8 Studies on sexual activity are notoriously difficult to carry out. Until the award of grants from the Medical Research Council and the Department of Health for Project Sigma (Socio-Sexual Investigations of Gay Men and AIDS) to a team of researchers chaired by Professor Tony Coxon, University of Wales, Cardiff (of which the author is a member), the only research team which would seem to have spent sufficient time on developing appropriate interviewing techniques to enable believable results to be obtained (Kinsey, Pomeroy and Martin, *Sexual Behaviour in the Human Male*, pp.35–62. See also note 8, ch. 3.
9 Child-adult sex is a subject which raises much emotion. Three useful books are Rossman, Rev P. *Sexual Experience between Men and Boys*, Maurice Temple Smith, 1985 (first published in the USA in 1976); O'Carroll, T. *Paedophilia: the Radical Case*, Owen, P. 1980 and Tsang, D. (ed) *The Age Taboo*, Alyson & GMP, 1981.
10 Useful insights are provided by the magazine *Trans*, and by

Kirk, K. and Heath, E. *Men in Frocks*, GMP, 1984.
11 Samaritans have operated a special system for callers of this type since 1973, known as the 'Brenda' system. Callers thought to be 'wankers' were referred to a special volunteer (or group of volunteers) known as 'Brenda'. Varah, *The Samaritans*, pp.148–161.
12 See note 15, ch. 3.

Chapter 7

1 See note 28, ch. 1.
2 However the policy adopted by the National Association of Citizens Advice Bureaux at its AGM in 1987 should provide a good example to other similar bodies.
3 See Williams, A. 'Swing to the Moral Right', *Marriage Guidance*, Autumn 1985, pp.2–5, '[The values of the] Moral Righters [are] middle class, religion-based and traditional in the sense that they are impervious to social change – a ludicrously restricted pattern to try to impose on our open pluralistic society.' (p.3) See also Weeks, J. *Sex, Politics and Society: The Regulation of Sexuality since 1800*, Longman, 1981, pp.279–282.
4 See Owen, D. 'Gay Rights and Social Democracy', *Gay Times*, April 1986 (91), pp.32–33 and Parker, J. 'No Going Back' in Cant and Hemmings, *Radical Records*, pp.259–266.

Index

Note: the words *advice, gay, heterosexual, identity, information, lesbian, sexual* are used throughout the book, and therefore are indexed only where a particular use requires it.

abuse, 26, 29–31
Acquired Immune Deficiency Syndrome *see* AIDS
advertising, 58, 59
advice never neutral, 3
for 'homosexuals; 8, 9
AIDS and HIV infection, xi, 12–14, 17, 39–43, 80, 97, 108, 125
and press hysteria, 12–13, 20
AIDS lines, 13, 17
Albany Trust, 11
Asian callers, 3, 10, 65

bereavement, 7
bisexuality, 34
black callers, 10, 65
Body Positive, 43

Campaign for Homosexual Equality, 10, 11, 85
cancer, 3
Capital Gay (newspaper), 21, 107
Chambers of Commerce, 48
charlatans, 52
Christian gay counselling services, 36n, 61
church, churches, 8, 36
Church of England, 14–15
clause 28, 14, 20, 29, 43, 85, 126
confidentiality, 23, 27–8
conformity, social, 82–4, 89–90

cottaging, 95–96
counselling
directive and non-directive, 60–63
quality of, 23, 119–22
cross-dressing, 99–103
custody of children, 75–8

datelines, 15–16
dating agencies, 104–5
directive *see* counselling,
'dirty talk', 108
discussions between volunteers as quality control, 120

empowerment, 10, 19–20
exploitation, 19–21

faithfulness in relationships *see* relationships
feminism
philosophy and ideas, 17, 18, 75, 103
FRIEND, iv, 11–12, 16, 17, 84, 122
Friends of the helpline, 121

Gay and Lesbian Professional Caucuses, 48, 49
gay helpline
definition, xii–xiii
functions of, 111–13

numbers of, xii
number of calls to, ii, xii
quality of, 119–122
reasons for existence, 7–10
Gay Liberation Front, 10, 85
gay liberation
 philosophy and ideas, 11, 75
Gay Life (magazine), 21, 107
gayline, xiv, 17
Gay News (newspaper), 11
Gay Scotland (magazine), 21, 107
Gay Sweatshop (theatre group), 81
Gay Switchboard, 4, 20
 see also Lesbian and Gay Switchboard
Gay Times (magazine), 21, 107
gender roles, 44–5
ghettos, 6, 18
Government (of the UK), 13, 14

Hall-Carpenter Archive, 81
helpline
 definition, xi
 gay *see* gay helpline
 specialist gay, 18
HIV infection *see* AIDS
Homosexual Law Reform Society, 11
homosexual
 use of word, xiii
homosexuality
 debates concerning causalities, 35–6
homophobia, 12–13
Human Immuno-deficiency Virus *see* AIDS

Icebreakers, 11
information agencies, 16, 112
interpreter, gay helplines as, 113–14
Islam, 35

Jewry, British, 35

Kinsey, Dr Alfred, 39, 99
Knight, Dame Jill MP *see* clause 28

Lambda Business Councils, 48, 49
legal profession, 1, 77–8, 95–6

Lesbian and Gay Christian Movement, 15, 36
Lesbian and Gay Switchboards, xiii, 11, 16–17, 56–7
Lesbian and Gay Switchboard, London, 11, 18, 56
library sevice, public, 114–15
Local Government Act, 1988 *see* clause 28
Local Government Bill *see* clause 28
London, Church of England Diocese of, 15

management of helplines, 57–58, 119–22
marriage
 arranged, 3
 counselling on, 65
 disclosures within, 74–78
masturbation calls, 107–9
medical profession, 1, 96–7
medical researchers, 35
mobility handicaps, persons with, 10, 64
monogamy, 78–82
multiple sclerosis, 70–1

normal
 'the normal 40–year old man', 36
non-directive *see* counselling
nightclubs, 85

parents, disclosures to, 68–74
Parliament, 8, 14
peer review as quality control, 122
Pink Paper, The (newspaper), 21, 107
police, 27, 95, 97–8
political change
 helplines as agents for, 3–4
press hysteria over AIDS *see* AIDS
Pride March, annual Lesbian and Gay, 21
'problem', 'homosexuality' as a, 8–9
'promotion of homosexuality' intentional *see* clause 28
'promiscuity', 40–1

psychiatry, psychiatrists, 8, 93–4
public accountabilility
  as quality control, 121
Public Service Announcements, 58
pubs, gay, 45–9, 84–5

quality of service, 119–22
'queer' as term of abuse, 29, 30

rape, 97–8
referees for volunteers, 54
referrals to other
  agencies, 91, 94–7
relationships
  faithfulness in, 78–82
  series of, 79
records for quality
  control, 120–121
role models, 78–79

safer sex, 42
Samaritans, 2, 5, 55, 116–18
secrecy, 28–9
selection of volunteers *see*
  volunteers
sensory handicaps, persons
  with, 10
Sexual Offences Act 1967, 10, 93
sexual techniques, 43–5
sexually transmitted diseases, 96–7
silence, 24–26

Smith, Chris MP, 14
social scientists, 35
spina bifida, 7
Stop the Clause Campaign, 85
support groups run by
  helplines, 58, 86–9
support for helplines, 27, 127
switchboards, xiv

teenagers' groups, gay, 87–9
Telecom, British, 15–16
Terrence Higgins Trust, 13, 40
theologians, 34–6
therapy, sex as, 105–6
trade unions, 13
training of volunteers *see*
  volunteers
transvestism, 91, 99–103

Varah, Rev Chad, 2
volunteering, 18–19, 51–7
volunteer bureau, 53
volunteers
  selection of, 51–5
  training of, 51–7, 66–7
  strains on, 74, 82
  professional help for, 98–9

Wilshire, David MP *see*
  clause 28
'wankers', 104, 107–9